The Power of Clan

The Power of Clan

The Influence of Human Relationships on Heart Disease

Stewart Wolf

John G. Bruhn

With the Collaboration of

Brenda P. Egolf
Judith Lasker
Billy U. Philips

Photographs by Remsen Wolff

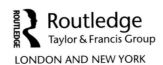

Routledge
Taylor & Francis Group

LONDON AND NEW YORK

First published 1993 by Transaction Publishers
First paperback edition 1998

Published 2019 by Routledge
2 Park Square, Milton Park, Abingdon, Oxon OX14 4RN
52 Vanderbilt Avenue, New York, NY 10017

Routledge is an imprint of the Taylor & Francis Group, an informa business

Library of Congress Catalog Number: 91-42290

Library of Congress Cataloging-in-Publication Data

Wolf, Stewart, 1914
The power of clan : the influence of human relationships on heart disease / Stewart Wolf, John G. Bruhn ; with the collaboration of Brenda P. Egolf, Judith N. Lasker, Billy U. Philips ; photographs by Remsen Wolff.
   p. cm.
   Includes index.
   ISBN 1-56000-043-0
   1. Heart—Infarction—Pennsylvania—Roseto—Mortality. 2. Coronary heart disease—Social aspects. 3. Health surveys—Pennsylvania—Roseto. 4. Roseto (Pa.)—Social life. 5. Italian Americans—Health and hygiene. 6. Italian Americans—Social life and customs. I. Bruhn, John G., 1934. II. Title.
RA645.H4W65   1992
616.1'23'0019—dc20   91-42290
                                    CIP

ISBN 13: 978-0-7658-0449-5 (pbk)
ISBN 13: 978-1-56000-043-3 (hbk)

Contents

Preface and Acknowledgments

A prospective study of the relationship of social adjustment to coronary heart disease in the Italian American town of Roseto, Pennsylvania, began 30 years ago. What has been learned seems to confirm an old but often forgotten conviction that mutual respect and cooperation contribute to the health and welfare of a community and its inhabitants, and that self-indulgence and lack of concern for others exert opposite influences.

This book is a sequel to one published in 1979. We are grateful to the University of Oklahoma Press, Norman, Oklahoma, for permission to revise and reproduce some material from the original volume.

Those who helped with the initial study of Roseto and its inhabitants and of the control communities in the vicinity of Roseto were acknowledged in the first book, The Roseto Story—An Anatomy of Health. The indispensable help of Florence Giaquinto and members of her family during the sociomedical survey should be reacknowledged, as should the skillful devoted administrative work of Mrs. James H. Ross.

The follow-up survey, beginning in 1985, was carried out in collaboration with the Center for Social Research at Lehigh University, Bethlehem, Pennsylvania, under the leadership of its director, Roy C. Herrenkohl, professor of social relations and now vice provost for research and dean of graduate studies. In 1986 the Lehigh group made house-to-house visits to families in Roseto and Bangor to conduct individual sociological interviews. Brenda Egolf implemented and supervised the data handling throughout the period 1985 to 1990. She, Judy Lasker, and Louise Potvin performed most of the work on mortality rates presented in chapter 5. Judy Lasker and Brenda Egolf researched and wrote up the data on social change in Roseto and Bangor that appear in chapter 8. Also from Lehigh University, Professor Donald T. Campbell has provided invaluable advice and counsel and has graciously shared his expertise and experience in research design and evaluation.

The other collaborating group was from the University of Texas Medical Branch in Galveston. Billy U. Philips, professor of preventive medicine and community health and associate dean of the College of Allied Health Sciences and his associate, Steve Shelton brought a corps of selected senior physician's-assistant students to assist with the individual interviews and physical examinations. They included Pamela Cruse (now Martocci), Howard and Emilie Brummett, Jim Sterling, and Deborah Wynder. The examinations were held at the same school building as before, which is now called the Faith Christian School. Judith Jones organized and operated the clinic with the assistance of her son Christopher Dentith, Ann Jeannette Ruggiero (now Peiffer), her sister Donna, and Melissa Bartosh, Ricky Ball, and Sandra Riggs, with invaluable volunteer assistance from Rosalyn Mugavero, and Mimi Trigiani, Mamie Cilibenti Lucille Guida, Pat Ronca, Al Ronca, Jean Anne D'Alessio, Antoinette Goffredo, Bill Counterman, and Tony DiPalma. The laboratory work was under the direction of Dr. Arthur Sevem assisted by Virginia Derbyshire, Sharon Hahn, Marie Koehler, and Jason Perry. Charmaine Cesare, Mary Detrick, Caroline Dunnachie and Paula Dahlenburg served as electrocardiographic technicians. Dr. Ragner Levi of the Karolinska Institute in Stockholm participated in all aspects of the work, and Dr. Alvin P. Shapiro, professor of medicine at the University of Pittsburgh, also participated and shared his clinical expertise. Assistance with data retrieval and statistical analysis was provided by Elbert Whorton and Jacob Ebey.

Editorial assistance was provided by Helen Goodell and Barbara Griffin. The graphs and some of the tables were executed by Camille Muhlbach, and Joy Lowe skillfully rendered the manuscript through multifold revisions.

The photographs by Remsen Wolff were supplemented with a few by Steve Shapiro and Tom Wolf. The stills from TV tapes in chapters 7 and 8 were reproduced with permission from Medstar Productions and Ellbe-TV-Ltd.

The research was supported by grants from the National Institute on Aging #1R0,1AG04957, the Eleanor Naylor Dana Charitable Trust, The Pew Charitable Trust, and the Kaiser Family Foundation.

We are grateful to Irving Louis Horowitz, president of Transaction Publishers and his wife, Mary Curtis, editor, for their frank and supportive criticism and suggestions and to Esther Luckett who skillfully shepherded the manuscript through the process of publication.

1

The Medical Significance
of the Social Environment

*There can be hope only for a society which acts as one
big family, and not as many separate ones.*
—Anwar Sadat[1]

The organization of early civilized communities was based on family
units. As families reproduced and enlarged, they developed into kinships,
or *clans*, a Gaelic word derived from the Latin scion. With more or less
common ancestry, a clan became an alliance, or mutually protective
brotherhood, with established standards of values and behavior. Clans
still exert powerful sociopolitical influence in many developing countries
and continue to symbolize an honored unifying tradition in such indus-
trialized areas as Scotland.

For many centuries, when the parts of the world remained isolated
from one another, clans with established traditions for successive leadership managed to maintain a considerable measure of social stability for
many years, although it was not unusual for nearby clans to war with one
another during one or two seasons of the year. When this practice was
held within limits, the interrelationships within a clan were actually
strengthened. With improved transportation, wider communication, and
more lethal instruments of war, however, the stability of the clan order
was threatened. Even more conducive to instability, it appears, was the
seductive intrusion of foreign social influences, a calamity that affected

community after community in the islands of the Pacific, South America, parts of Africa and elsewhere throughout the world as European explorers sought to introduce their ways of life.

In 1938 in a book entitled *Civilization and Disease*, C.P. Donnison, who had worked for many years as a physician in black Africa, reported that he had encountered no hypertension, diabetes or peptic ulcer in remote areas of the continent where the prevailing social structure was relatively stable.[2] These and other chronic diseases did appear, however, where "civilizing" forces were rapidly invading an established culture.

W. L. Brown, in his introduction to Donnison's perceptive monograph, states in his first sentence, "Physically, the evolution of Man appears to be at a standstill, and it would be a bold man who would maintain that mentally there has been an advance since the days of the ancient Greeks. It is on the psychological side, by which man adjusts himself to his environment, that we can alone expect [advances] to be made."[3]

Donnison's book develops the idea that, as man has lived in groups of increasing size, social patterns have evolved to deal with prevailing challenges, and that over the course of history and in various parts of the world, social structures have been altered and remodeled to meet changing circumstances. Donnison suggests that when the speed of change has outrun the pace of adaptation, man's internal mechanisms, mental and physical, acting inappropriately, provide what he calls the basis of the diseases of civilization.

Ten years after Donnison's book appeared, J. L. Halliday in England picked up the idea of the potential pathogenicity of social forces and wrote a book called *Psychosocial Medicine*.[4] Halliday argued that although it was obvious to everyone that attention to the physical environment had made possible some of the most effective public health measures—the control of typhoid fever, cholera, plague, typhus, and other infectious diseases, and more recently the control of radiation and of pathogenic chemicals in the environment—similar concern with the psychological and social environment, however appropriate, had lagged behind.

Both Donnison and Halliday saw morale, or common purpose, as the healthy integrating force in society. They both considered disease the consequence of demoralization related to social change, change too swift or too disruptive for the adaptive capacity of the social group.

L. W. Simmons and Harold G. Wolff, dealing with this issue in their book *Social Science in Medicine*,[5] observed that in decaying cultures anxiety-producing factors tend to outlast those that protect against or relieve anxiety. Similarly, René Dubos showed that vulnerability to infectious diseases may be enhanced in a setting of rapid social change.[6] After a lifetime of study of tuberculosis, he concluded that unsanitary conditions, crowding, poverty, and so forth were less significant in outbreaks of the disease throughout the world than what he referred to as "social disruption," or rapid social change. Many other scientists have added confirmation to the concept that the quality of social adaptation is pertinent to health. Indeed, this basic proposition has cropped up repeatedly since antiquity. Nevertheless, it is still not wholly acceptable to the biomedical community, and has yet to be incorporated in currently prevailing thought about medicine and public health, which has been largely focused on the individual as the "unit of analysis," with very little attention given to the possible influence of group processes.

While it is the individual who either gets sick and dies or doesn't, and while individual genetic disposition is an important consideration in assessing the likelihood of a disease, the fact that there are striking differences in the prevalence of many diseases (myocardial infarction, for example) from time to time in the same country and from place to place on the globe strongly suggests inquiry into the social environment. Nevertheless, current emphasis in research has been on individual behaviors chiefly involving food, exercise, and smoking. These and other "risk factors" such as the serum concentration of cholesterol, alpha and beta lipoprotein, and triglycerides, together with coincident hypertension and diabetes, have been the main concerns of the long prospective study of Framingham, Massachusetts, where little attention has been accorded the possible influence of social forces in family and community.[7]

Also focused on the individual have been investigations of the possible contribution of temperament and personality to susceptibility of coronary heart disease. All of the above approaches have been productive, although they have not included inquiry into the influence of the social environment on individual behaviors and temperaments. The protective effect of certain temperamental characteristics such as "hardiness" and a "sense of coherence" has served to some extent to shift the emphasis from the individual to what has influenced the individual. Other investigators have turned their attention to the potentially pathogenic challenge of change and the physiological consequences of various adaptive or coping responses.[8-11] Interest in social influences has also been accelerated by the work of Lynch[12] on the damaging effects of loneliness, and of Karasek, Theorell, and Schwartz[13] on the risk of coronary heart disease among workers in jobs that make strong demands but offer little opportunity for them to control their way of meeting those demands. The medical significance of social forces has also been evident in several studies showing that even after controlling for the established behavioral risk factors, social activities and relationships play a crucial role in susceptibility to coronary disease.[14,15]

Studies of populations undergoing rapid social change suggest that the change itself, apart from behavioral correlates, may be sufficiently stressful to create an increase in vulnerability to disease. These studies, and especially those of Cassel have caused a reawakening of interest in the earlier work of Donnison and others referred to above.[16] Recent advances in the understanding of the brain circuitry involved in responding to life experience discussed in chapter 8 of this book have revived an awareness of the role of sensation in homeostasis. It is therefore becoming easier to accept the proposition that perturbation of an established system may set in motion a destructive chain of events. Thus, an organism adapted to past circumstances may be to some extent maladapted to new ones. Brunner and his colleagues studied Oriental Jews who were immigrating to Israel and found that shortly after arrival they had low concentrations of serum cholesterol and practically no heart attacks.[17] Moreover, those who died in the early years following immigration showed at autopsy very little arteriosclerosis in their coronary vessels. Several years later, however, Brunner observed that the cholesterol concentration in Oriental Jews had risen, and they had begun to experience coronary artery disease, myocardial infarction (heart attack), and sudden death in increasing numbers. He pointed to the extraordinarily rapid social change that they had experienced.

The Oriental Jew, living in a tent in the desert in Africa with his wife and children, was accustomed to being the absolute ruler of the family. Suddenly in Israel his children were thrown into school, where they associated with peer groups that emphasized, as they do in this country, "doing your own thing" and freedom. At home, therefore, instead of showing their former automatic deference and respect to their fathers, they expressed themselves freely and were often rebellious. The wife and mother, who in the desert had been covered up literally and figuratively, could now exploit her skills at sewing and cooking, land a job, and earn money. On the job, surrounded by the ambience of women's lib, she might sometimes defy her husband. The frustration of the head of the household who possessed no marketable skills led, not surprisingly, to serious disequilibrium among these Oriental Jewish families in their new environment.

The European common market has provided another interesting laboratory for the study of the pathologic effects of radical social change. Uehlinger found that while Italians living in Italy had a very low incidence of myocardial infarction, the rate was higher among Italians working in Germany and was approaching that of their German comrades.[18] It may be that the Italians were now eating a richer fare, but it does not seem likely that diet could have increased the occurrence of myocardial infarction in so short a time. On the other hand, the stress of adjusting to radical and rapid social change may have had some relevance.

Similar observations were made by Seguin in South America. While studying the industrial setting in Lima, Peru, he found that the workers, displaced from the rural areas in the mountains to Lima, not only had more heart disease but more disease of all kinds than did their neighbors back home.[19]

A few years ago in the jungles of Brunei, Borneo, a situation reminiscent of Donnison's experience in Africa was observed.[20] During a period of rapid social change, diabetes, coronary disease, and hypertension, formerly rare, had begun to affect the inhabitants of the city. The rural tribes, however, who had held tenaciously to their centuries-old social customs, their communal living patterns in longhouses, and their animistic religion, had remained unaffected by these diseases despite the incursions of modern civilization. Since World War II, Brunei had been undergoing drastic changes brought on by its new riches from the discovery of offshore oil. Even in the rural areas, major social changes stemming from the availability of jobs in the oil and lumber industries or on the crews building roads that penetrated deeply into the jungle were taking place. Modern medicine was brought to every community by helicopter, and public health programs had virtually eliminated most tropical and other infectious diseases. Perhaps the most striking change of all was that schools had sprung up everywhere. It is too early to predict whether or not the healthy tribes of Borneo will ultimately succumb to the metabolic and vascular diseases so familiar to us. They should be studied prospectively as a younger generation emerges, a generation that may discard the sustaining traditional beliefs and the established way of life of their parents.

An opportunity to make such a prospective study was available much closer to home in the form of an experiment of nature in Roseto, an Italian community in eastern Pennsylvania.[21] We found that this community, which had clung to its "Old World" culture since immigration in 1882 and until the mid-1960s, had enjoyed relative freedom from heart attacks. In fact, the death rate from heart attack in Roseto was less than half that in neighboring communities, although the prevalence of usually accepted risk factors for heart attacks—consumption of animal fats, smoking, lack of exercise, hypertension, and diabetes—was at least as great in Roseto as in neighboring towns, where more than twice as many heart attacks were occurring and where the death rate from heart attack was similar to that of the United States at large.

Roseto in Perspective

In 1965 Daniel Romano, a native of Roseto, published a biography of his friend Peter Ronca who, he felt, embodied the spirit and traditions of Roseto.[22] Peter, a blacksmith and also a native of Roseto, had often declared: "I've got to work 'till I die.' He ultimately did exactly as he had said and died a blacksmith at the age of 94. Until the very day of his death he had been in constant demand for shoeing horses from racing stables all over the east coast. Peter, a perfectionist in his craft, was also one of the founders of Roseto's Roman Catholic church, a volunteer fireman, a part-time policeman, a champion of education, and a neighbor constantly helping those in trouble. His shop was a magnet to the children of Roseto. As mentioned above, his biographer believed that Peter embodied the essence of Roseto, a town where the family, not the individual, was seen as the unit of society, where an attitude of cooperation outpaced that of competition, and where greeting, enjoying, and helping neighbors was the order of the day.

The message of Roseto is not new, but it is unusually vivid. It suggests that both the personal and the more broadly social quality of human relationships are strikingly relevant to the health and longevity of human beings, especially with respect to coronary artery disease and sudden arrhythmic death. The evidence derives from a prospective study of this relatively homogeneous community of 1,600 in eastern Pennsylvania owned and operated by Italian immigrants and inhabited by them and their descendants for over 100 years.[21]

Roseto was settled in 1882 by Italians from Roseto Val Fortore, a town in southern Italy near the Adriatic Sea. The new community in the United States was established on one of the foothills of the Appalachian Mountains just east of the Delaware Water Gap, a setting much like that of their former home in Italy, which is located on the foothills of the Appenine Mountains in the Province of Foggia. For the past twenty-five years the community of Roseto, Pennsylvania, has been under more or less continuous observation as a laboratory for the study of the relationship of social change to health and longevity.

The Early Days

On their arrival in the United States, the Italian settlers found jobs in the slate quarries of Bangor, Pennsylvania, where two decades earlier immigrants from Bangor, North Wales, had settled and established the slate industry. The Welsh proprietors of the slate quarries treated the Italians badly, gave them the hardest and most dangerous jobs, and paid them very little. The Rosetans, inherently clannish, grew more so in the face of social exclusion and exploitation by their Welsh neighbors and employers.

Hardship and threats to existence were nothing new to southern Italians, however. As described in chapter 2, the émigrés from Roseto Val Fortore brought with them to America their long tradition of coping through 800 years of invasions by the Byzantines, Normans, Burgundians, Flemish, French, Spanish, Hungarians, Austrians, Germans, and Arabs, as well as warfare among Italy's city states. Luigi Barzini, in his book *The Italians*, tells of the turmoil that began when Charles VIII subdued the state of Naples at the battle of Fornovo, July 1495.[23] "Even the diligent old *Encyclopaedia Britannica*, wrote Barzini, 'groaned under the burden of having to clarify subsequent events to its readers and gave up.' Its 11th edition sadly says: 'it is impossible in this place to follow the tangled intrigues of the period.'"[24] Despite the protracted political chaos, Italy during those years of change produced some of the world's greatest art, music, literature, and scientific discoveries.

The book *Roseto Val Fortore*, published in 1971 by a one-time native, Msgr. Annibale Facchiano, chronicles the events during this period and the later confusion leading up to the unification of Italy.[25] He dwells on the remarkable resilience of the Rosetans in coping with a long string of conquerors and local rulers. As he put it: Legitimate heirs and conceited pretenders, vicious princesses, and weak princes, presumptuous knights and intransigent dignitaries clashed, squabbled and alternated in the exercise of power. They disfigured the dignity of royal power and broke up the order in public life. The people naturally paid the bill for this seemingly endless political mess through fiscal tributes, stealings of adventurers, and the breaking up of the faith and customs of the people.[25"] The ability of the paisani to maintain their values and carry on in the face of repeated turmoil recalls a comment in W. H. Auden's introduction to Goethe's *Italian Journey*: "Is there any other country in Europe where the character of the people seems to have been so little affected by political and technological change?"[26]

What did not change was their family solidarity and community cohesion. Barzini's book documents these powerful features of the Italian culture that seem to afford them the resilience to cope with an often hostile, rapidly changing environment.[23] The same family and community cohesion, together with shared traditions and religious devotion, distinguished Roseto, Pennsylvania, from the surrounding communities.[27] When immigrants began arriving in the late 1800s and up to the decade following World War I, they underwent serious hardships, social exclusion, and indignities at the hands of English and Welsh quarry owners. The English and the Welsh considered the skilled jobs their peculiar prerogative because their ancestors, having learned the slater's trade in the British Isles, were "qualified." The Italians were considered only good enough to "work in the hole or throw out the rubbish." They were paid only every three months at the rate of eight cents an hour for a ten-hour day and were required to shop at the company stores. These abuses stimulated them to establish their own enclave and look out for their own welfare, exploiting to the fullest the traditional tendency of Italians to maintain close family and community ties.

The Roseto Study

Our interest in Roseto was aroused in 1961 by a chance meeting with a local physician, Dr. Benjamin Falcone, who had noted that coronary artery disease was uncommon among Rosetans compared to the inhabitants of the immediately adjacent town of Bangor. Dr. Falcone's practice came from both communities. His observation stimulated us to study mortality records for Roseto and several nearby towns covering the seven-year period 1955-1961. We soon learned that the death rate from heart attack among men in Roseto had been less than half that of predominantly Welsh Bangor, nearby Nazareth, which was mainly ethnically German, ethnically mixed Stroudsburg and East Stroudsburg, and the United States at large (Figure 1.1).

FIGURE 1.1

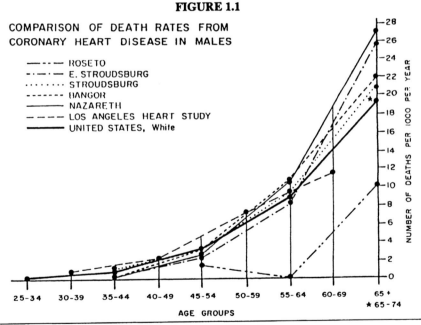

Comparison of Death Rates in Men from Myocardial Infarction

In an effort to determine the reasons for Roseto's remarkable immunity from fatal heart attack, we next undertook a systematic study of the inhabitants in Roseto and, for comparison, two neighboring communities, Bangor and Nazareth. We found that clinical evidence of coronary artery disease was significantly lower in Roseto than in the two neighboring control towns despite similar prevalence of conventional risk factors, including high serum cholesterol, high fat diet, and smoking. Figure 1.1 compares the death rate in Roseto from 1955 to 1961 with the rates in the control towns, Los Angeles, and the white population of the United States. To explain the discrepancy, we considered the possibility that Rosetan immigrants had come from especially sturdy stock not susceptible to coronary disease. That explanation appeared unlikely, however, when we were able to examine and interview members of Roseto families who lived elsewhere but returned to Roseto for a few days each year for the annual festival of Our Lady of Mt. Carmel, the town's most important celebration in which a tradition initiated in Roseto Val Fortore was carried over to the new world. The data on coronary disease among the relatives of Rosetans living elsewhere were similar to the findings of the control communities, Welsh Bangor, and German Nazareth. These studies, which involved individual detailed history, physical examination, electrocardiogram, blood chemistry, dietary, smoking, and drinking histories, and structured sociological interviews, have been published and summarized in *The Roseto Story: An Anatomy of Health.*[21]

Not only were the usually acknowledged risk factors for coronary disease at least as prevalent in Roseto as in the surrounding towns, but so were the familiar interpersonal family and occupational stresses. Roseto differed from the control communities, however, in terms of strong social support reflected in unusually close family ties and community cohesion. It appeared that the accustomed social behavior of Rosetans may have served to counteract stress since, as pointed out, their way of life emphasized cooperation and sharing rather than competition. The town radiated a kind of joyous team spirit as its inhabitants celebrated religious festivals and family landmarks such as birthdays, graduations, and engagements. Their social focus was on the family, whereas neighboring communities, holding to the traditional American view, were more likely to focus on the individual as the unit of society.

When we interviewed and examined the inhabitants of Roseto and familiarized ourselves with the town and its people, we were surprised at our inability to distinguish by dress, manner, or speech the affluent owners of textile factories from the more impecunious laborers. The well-kept houses of all Rosetans, rich and poor, were clustered close together on streets with colorful Italian names such as Dante, Columbus, and Garibaldi. The lack of display of affluence or even obvious distinction between rich and poor, and the absence of the need to "keep up with the Joneses" appeared to be a central ingredient in the unifying cohesive force of the community. We learned that it had its origin in the dim past of feudal or prefeudal Italy, mainly from the myth of *maloccio*, the evil eye. The belief was that any ostentation or display of superiority over one's neighbor would be punished by ill fortune.

The remarkable way of life in Roseto has been chronicled in several newspaper and magazine articles in this country including *McClure's Magazine* in 1908,[28] and the San Francisco Chronicle,[29] and in Italian American publications.[30] In recent years five television documentaries based on the Roseto Study have been made and shown in the United States, Sweden, and the United Kingdom. There have also been several books about Roseto. Apart from the biographical sketch of Peter Ronca referred to earlier, a short history of Roseto, was published in 1952 by a native, Ralph Basso.[31] Facchiano's book provides a scholarly archeological and historical account of his native town, beginning in the pre-Roman era and continuing through the unification of Italy and the emigration to Roseto, Pennsylvania.[25]

During the period of our original studies of Roseto, a graduate student in social anthropology at the University of Pennsylvania, Clement L. Valletta, was developing his doctoral thesis dealing with the social structure of the town, "The Settlement of Roseto: World View and Promise"[32] He later enlarged the work, changed the name of the town and the names of the families mentioned, and published it under the title *A Study of Americanization in Carneta.*[33]

Meanwhile in 1974 Carla Bianco, a professor of anthropology at the Rome branch of Temple University, published *The Two Roseto's*, which compared the folklore beliefs and practices of Roseto Val Fortore with the Pennsylvania Roseto.[34] She began her work in Roseto, Pennsylvania, during the period of our original study. Her book and the other three works cited emphasize for Roseto, as Barzini did for Italians in general, the contribution of family cohesion to the strength and stability of communities.

We will attempt in this book to document the changes in Roseto and its people that have occurred as they have adapted to life in the United States, and to test the hypothesis that community morale and individual commitment to family and tradition are conducive to health. The book will also examine the obverse, that is, evidence of the pathogenic potential of change and ambiguity in the social environment.

2

Roseto's History: Turmoil, Cohesion, and Adaptation

As mentioned in the previous chapter, most of the inhabitants of Roseto, Pennsylvania, trace their origin to a hill town in Southern Italy located at a level of about 2,200 feet in the foothills of the Appenine Mountains near the Adriatic coast. According to the historian Msgr. Annibale Facchiano, the area was occupied by four ancient tribes before the days of the Roman Empire: the Sanniti, the Frentani, the Irpini, and the Dauni.[25] The precise location that became Roseto was in the area occupied by the Sanniti, who called their territory Sannio. It is said that linguists have been able to identify elements of the language of the Sanniti in the dialect of Roseto. Moreover, there is historical evidence, based partly on the geographical characteristics of the land, that the ethnic group that settled Roseto, the Sanniti, continued to live there during the era of the Roman Empire.

During the Punic Wars (218-202 B.C.) and after the battle of Trasimeno (217 B.C.) Hannibal invaded and occupied Sannio and the province of Daunia, which later became known as Foggia. He then devastated Sannio because the inhabitants had remained faithful to the Romans. In A.D. 1000 during the period of the Byzantine Empire, the region where Roseto was located was crisscrossed by armies during the fighting against the Normans and the Germanic tribes. In 1019, the Byzantines defeated the Normans on the plain of Canne. At that time the name *Roseto* was apparently applied to a cluster of houses in the region,

13

but the name had not as yet been applied to a town until later in the Eleventh century by the members of a prominent family named Falcone. Nine centuries later Lorenzo Falcone, with two others from Roseto Val Fortore, founded the village of New Italy, which later became Roseto, Pennsylvania.

According to the historian V. A. LaPenna, the original inhabitants of Roseto gathered there from three places in the region known as Ripa, Vetruscelli, and Rocchetta. The founders described it as a place dear and romantic, where shrubs of fragrant wild roses were blooming and where a little old church dedicated to St. Lappiano was still maintained. The Ruggiero family,* also from Ripa, soon arrived to be joined by the Rinaldis, the Capobiancos, the Zitos, and the LaPennas, as well as other families whose names are familiar in Roseto, Pennsylvania, today.

The strategic importance of the area was attested to by the number of castles built there by the Normans, the Byzantines, and the Longobards. Roseto appears to have been an important defensive base for the regional leader of the Byzantine army, Captain Bogiano.

The Byzantines were able to savor their triumph for only a little over half a century when the Normans resumed the war, ultimately defeated the Byzantines, and went on to unify the entire area of southern Italy and Sicily under Robert II (Guiscardo), who died in 1085. His oldest son, Ruggero, duke of Calabria, was invested as king in 1100 by Pope Pasquale II. Control over the entire area was difficult to maintain, however, against local counts and dukes who continually contended for dominion. In 1122 a count named Giordano succeeded in occupying Roseto and its surroundings, after which a truce established by Pope Callisto II held for a time.

Ruggero was succeeded by his son, Ruggero II, grandson of Guiscardo. He tried to regain the Roseto region but was excommunicated by the pope in 1127. Ten years later, however, Ruggero II was able to resume his position as ruler of all of Sicily and southern Italy, allowing a local nobleman, Guillelmo Potofranco, to govern Roseto.

Eventually the Norman monarchy fell, and Frederick II of the Hohenstauffen family, who in 1220 had been crowned Holy Roman Emperor, took dominion over southern Italy and Sicily. He brought in Saracens to guard the area, and although they were stationed in the nearby

---

*   Members of this family were also among the earliest settlers of Roseto, Pennsylvania.

town of Lucera which quickly took on a Muslim character, Roseto was apparently unaffected by the Saracen presence or its influence.

Frederick, who had hoped also to conquer northern Italy with the help of his Saracen army, found himself continually in conflict with the Pope who excommunicated him and repeatedly accepted him back into the church. Frederick's death in 1250 brought on another period of conflict and confusion, with fighting between the Saracens and the Germans. In 1265 Pope Urban IV appealed to the French king, Louis IX (St. Louis). He sent his brother Charles, count of Anjou (Angio), who within five years had conquered the Germans and the Saracens and established himself as Charles I, king of Naples.

Roseto suffered severely, and may have been uninhabited for a time during the reign of Charles I, who was constantly at war with Peter III of Aragon and others. Charles I died in Foggia in 1285 and was succeeded by his son, Charles II who in 1294 assigned the fiefdom of Roseto to Bartolomeo Di Capua, giving him the task of rebuilding the place and reestablishing the community. In 1338 Charles's son Roberto of Angio further enlarged the fiefdom with more land and more people from the nearby encampment of Ventruscelli.

In 1443 King Alphonso V of Aragon, whose predecessors had conquered Sicily, established Spanish rule in Italy by becoming king of Naples. He was succeeded in 1458 by his son Ferdinand I, but the Di Capua family held on at Roseto. Bartolomeo Di Capua III built the parochial church and the baronial palace while other feudal lords in the region continued their fighting. Despite the turmoil, the period was a relatively happy and productive one for Roseto, which remained under the feudal rule of the Di Capua family from 1294 to 1556, when Giovanni Di Capua sold Roseto to Fernando Lombardo of Troia for 24,000 ducats. Thereafter, Roseto was buffeted about as the prize of warring noble families.

The confusing era of the wars between France and Spain ensued until the Treaty of Blois in 1504-1505 gave Sicily and Naples to Spain. High taxes and other oppression were visited on the Rosetans for most of the next 200 years. By the mid-seventeenth century the Brancia family had become the owners of Roseto. In 1655 they sold the town to Baron Giuseppe Saggese of Foggia for 49,500 ducats. Five generations of the Saggese family ruled Roseto for the next hundred years during which Roseto endured one calamity after another: the bubonic plague and two eruptions of Vesuvius. There was a large mortality from repeated famines endured under the despotic regime of the Spanish rulers of the kingdom of Naples. After the French Revolution the Spanish-French conflict resumed, displacing one ruler after the other including Joseph Bonaparte, brother of Napoleon I, who reigned for two years. But ultimately the Spanish Bourbons were restored and ruled until 1860, when Naples was annexed to Sardinia.

The Nineteenth Century

The revolution of 1848 touched Italy, as it did most of the rest of Europe, with a revolt against Bourbon rule which in Roseto was led by the six Capobianco brothers.* The unification of Italy was in preparation. Many of Roseto's families were politically active during this period on both sides of the conflict.

As Facchiano tells it, "commanding a mutinous and tumultuous band, they forced Vincenzo Falcone, who had become a supporter of the Bourbon king, to renounce his job as mayor." (Michael Falcone is currently mayor of Roseto, Pennsylvania). The Capobianco home was searched and their mother, D. Orazio Scrocca, who had been roughed up, maintained her dignity and courage and, according to Facchiano, "did not abandon her austere reserve." On July 17, 1850, the Capobianco brothers were arrested but were never prosecuted. The population of Roseto remained divided between those who were loyal to the Bourbon king and those who favored the unification of Italy under King Victor Emanuel. There were many local battles. Several of those still loyal to the Bourbons were captured and executed by a firing squad.

Following the unification of Italy as a monarchy with a democratic system, rival political parties appeared. In Roseto the more affluent and those who had been favorable to the Bourbon regime lived in a part of town with a higher elevation and were hence called the higher party, while the less affluent, who were more committed to liberal ideas, were called the lower party. Members of the higher party included the Falcones; the dominant family in the lower party were the Capobiancos. Although the two parties contrasted sharply in their political views, there was absolutely no bar to intermarriage among families belonging to the two parties.

---

*   Members of the Capobianco family have traditionally been among the most politically active of Roseto, Pennsylvania.

Following unification, the breakup of the big estates and the assignment of lots to families began and, not surprisingly, caused a great deal of turmoil among the inhabitants of Roseto, whose population had reached 5,000. There was widespread discontent, fueled by a prolonged poverty resulting from the dislocations of the wars of unification.

The villagers were especially receptive to the tales of riches and the "good life" in America. By 1882 the first wave of emigrants from Roseto had sailed to New York, encouraged by enthusiastic letters written by a Jesuit priest from Baltimore, Luigi Sabetti. Father Sabetti, a native of Roseto, was the posthumous son and fifteenth child of the town's doctor. In 1849, when he was ten years old, his mother died. Unwilling to be a financial burden to his older siblings, the young boy was determined to become a Jesuit priest. After schooling in Naples and France, he was ordained to the priesthood in 1868. Three years later he sailed for the United States, where he joined Woodstock College in Maryland as professor of moral theology.

Father Sabetti's letters to family and friends in Roseto encouraged many to want to emigrate to America. United States immigration laws at that time were nonrestrictive, and the passage to America was relatively inexpensive. The Italian authorities, however, considered emigration unpatriotic and at first declined permission to the Rosetans and a few other would-be emigrants from the nearby villages of Biccari, Castelluccio, Valmaggiore, and Alberona.[33] After the local authorities finally relented, thanks to the persuasive efforts of several influential people, the first group of eleven Rosetans, ten men and one boy (joined by three men and one boy from Castelfranco), left Italy in January 1882 for New York.[26] One of the steamer's passengers died from an infectious disease during the voyage, causing everyone to be quarantined for one month.[34] When the passengers were finally allowed to disembark, the Rosetan travelers went directly to the Italian settlement on Mulberry Street, where they spent the night on the tavern floor. An Italian railroad contractor, exacting a commission of one dollar from each of them, promised them work in Perth Amboy, New Jersey. The offer turned out to be a swindle, but eventually they obtained employment through a New York City employment agency: three as carpenters in Polatka, Florida, and eight as slate-quarry laborers in Howell Town, Pennsylvania, now part of Bangor.

The following year several more immigrants from Roseto managed to reach Howell Town, where they, too, became slate-quarry laborers. They worked hard and saved their money so that they might bring their relatives over from Italy.[26] All the new arrivals were men until Lorenzo Falcone arrived with his wife and two young children in 1884. Their next two children-a girl, Anna, and a boy, Anthony-became the first girl and the first boy to be born in Roseto which the immigrants originally called New Italy. Altogether, they had six daughters and five sons. Soon Lorenzo's brother, Ralph, arrived with his bride, a sister of Lorenzo's wife. It is perhaps not surprising that during our study of Roseto we learned that nearly two-thirds of the population was related by blood or marriage to the Falcones.

The immigrants established their community on a hillside tract that was linked to adjacent Bangor only by a rough wagon road and the tracks of the Central Railroad of New Jersey, which crossed it from north to south. The land could be bought cheaply and with little formality because its trees had been stripped and sold for lumber. Only rubbish, stumps, and stones remained; nevertheless, lots were bought and houses built. As described by Valletta, immigrants ingeniously used available materials: native stone for building, slate roofs, walls, and walks.[32] They helped each other dig out and build stone foundations for houses that were initially four-room, one-story, stone structures. There were no privately owned stores at first, no druggists or doctors. In 1892 the New Italy Hotel was opened by the first naturalized citizen, Lorenzo Pacifico. He sold wine, beer, and liquor in addition to tickets for transoceanic trips. The travel money was handled through an Italian bank in New York City. Grocery stores and other shops soon opened in Roseto. The community continued to grow as a steady stream of new immigrants arrived from Italy. Those days were marked by much confusion, competition, fights, and even petty crime among the settlers.

The older immigrants attributed their unrest to the absence of religious support and authority. The nearest Roman Catholic church was in Easton, Pennsylvania, nearly 20 miles away. With the hope of a place to worship closer to home, Archbishop Ryan, the Roman Catholic bishop of Philadelphia, was petitioned to establish a mission church in New Italy. He declined to do so. In 1887 Michelangelo D'Uva, who had been converted to Protestantism, visited New Italy with another Italian convert, Giovanni Gozzolino. D'Uva had come to the United States with Dr. Cardo, a physician who had helped several immigrants from Roseto Val Fortore get to America and had found them jobs in Amsterdam, New York. D'Uva and Gozzolino went from house to house in New Italy distributing free copies of the bible and religious pamphlets in the Italian language. Soon the villagers of New Italy were attending a Presbyterian church at Five Points, only five miles from home, where there happened to be an Italian pastor, the Reverend A. Arrhigi.

Rev. Arrhigi took a great interest in the immigrants and helped them in many ways, finally managing to persuade the presbytery to open an evangelical mission in New Italy. The Italians were able to recruit as their first pastor a Lombard Waldensian priest, Emmanual Tealdo. The first services were held in a shanty with boards laid across for pews and an empty beer keg as a pulpit. There were special services in English on Tuesday afternoons to help the congregation with the language. In addition, evening services featured talks by missionaries who worked in other Italian settlements in the United States. In 1893, with D'Uva's financial assistance, the members constructed a one-room building on a plot of land donated by one of the converts.[35] Thus the Presbyterian mission was chartered with sixty-four members. Later on in 1908 a few discontented Presbyterians joined the Jehovah's Witnesses and built a Kingdom Hall on Garibaldi Avenue. Eventually the growth of the sect made it necessary to build a new and larger Kingdom Hall on the main highway.

Those who still considered themselves Roman Catholics mounted the first religious celebration of the Festival of Mt. Carmel in 1889, with an Augustinian priest from Philadelphia who said the mass on an improvised alter near the house of Roseto's first citizen, Lorenzo Falcone. The following year they were able to recruit a Neapolitan priest from New York City. In the absence of a church, however, and a statue of the Blessed Virgin, the celebration had to be considered secular. The desire to build their own Catholic church became more urgent for the faithful, but the various families could not agree on where to locate it. Each family wanted it to be near its house. Finally, thanks to the generosity of the heads of the several families, a Catholic church dedicated to our Lady of Mt. Carmel was built in 1893 and completed the following year, a few days before the completion of the Protestant church. Its establishment stemmed the tide of conversions to Protestantism, but since no priest was available to provide full-time service, the church remained mostly closed for the next three years, with the Catholics attending St. Bernard's Church in Easton.

Meanwhile, Ralph Basso, author of *A History of Roseto* organized the Mutual Aid Society of St. Philip Neri to teach the catholic religion and American customs.[31] The community was now prepared to mount a truly ecclesiastical festival dedicated to Our Lady of Mt. Carmel in the traditional fashion carried over from Roseto Val Fortore in Italy. What became an annual celebration from then on was inaugurated during the last week of July 1894. Masses were said by priests from Philadelphia and New York, who blessed the Italian and American flags in a special ceremony. Classical Italian music was provided by two brass bands, the Roma Band of Philadelphia and the Bersagliere Band of New York. The festival attracted vast crowds both Italian and American, from surrounding towns. Many visitors—enchanted by the town's peaceful surroundings, fresh spring water from the Blue Mountains, and Italian food—chose to spend their summer vacations in the region. Others, including Italian shoemakers, blacksmiths, barbers, and tailors, deserted New York and Philadelphia to open their shops in nearby communities.

Finally, in 1896, Archbishop Ryan reversed his decision to deny the residents of New Italy their missionary church. He managed to recruit an Italian priest, Father Pasquale de Nisco, from a parish in London, England, to establish a full-time mission in New Italy. Father de Nisco, a cultured and sophisticated man, found a disorganized, dispirited group of Italian immigrants clinging to their land but knowing little English and nearly nothing about their adopted country. There was no coordination of effort, no appreciation of the responsibilities of citizenship. Some who had come with the early waves of immigration, ten or more years before, were fairly well established in the community and had started businesses. Other more recent arrivals were restive, bewildered, resentful, and sometimes seriously disruptive.

Father de Nisco quickly assumed leadership in the community. He bought twenty-eight lots at the top of the hill where the church of Our Lady of Mt. Carmel had been built which had had no assigned priest. He exhorted the Italian Presbyterians to return to their mother church or face excommunication. Working by himself with pick and shovel, he began to create a park and a cemetery. To encourage the inhabitants to do likewise, he bought and gave away flower seeds and bulbs and offered prizes for the best flower garden. Soon every foot of land was spaded and planted with flowers or vegetables, so that when in 1908 Marion Carter, a writer for *McClure's Magazine*, arrived from New York to report on Roseto, she saw

> a prosperous, lively little town, with dwelling-houses of good American clapboards and pale pressed brick, and with stores along its main street—groceries, markets, dry goods, and millinery stores; a druggist's shop, a hotel, a "Banca Italiana," a factory, a church on top of a hill with a mast-high flagpole and an American flag that marks out the spot for miles away; and gardens and gardens, and then more gardens, all with grape arbors; and when apparently one has come to the end of everything, a few more gardens tucked under a hillside. It is the garden aspect that first takes hold of one's imagination when one comes to Roseto. Of this town, which contains today more than two thousand inhabitants, Father de Nisco is *de facto* mayor, building inspector, health department, and arbiter of all questions relating to social conditions or business undertakings. He is also the chief of the police force, the president of the labor union, the founder of most of the clubs—social, literary, musical, theatrical, benevolent— and the organizer of the famous brass band, pride of Roseto and envy of the surrounding country, and of the baseball nine, whose husky youths affectionately declare that he can umpire a game better than anyone else.[28]

Father de Nisco's emphasis on beautification, learning English, becoming American, participating in politics, and especially the importance of education, together with his insistence on traditional Italian concern for the family, the church, and community pride, was unrelenting. He inaugurated a comprehensive plan for public improvement that was to serve as a pattern for subsequent progress. He encouraged his parishioners to secure American citizenship, urged parents to send their children to school, established clubs to promote interest in sports, initiated a circulating library, and formed organizations to meet the spiritual needs of specific age groups. The Mutual Aid Society, Addolorata, looked after the spiritual welfare of adults; the San Luigi Society worked among boys; the Sacred Heart Sodality was directed to mothers and wives; and the Figlie de Maria promoted Christian life among girls.

Father de Nisco began a campaign in the pulpit, in homes, and in the country court against "Sicilianism." His efforts were effective in reducing petty lawlessness. Most lawbreakers either reformed or left the area. He emphasized the need for cleanliness, often supervising the removal of trash and urging residents to improve their housing. Land values doubled nearly every two years, and the average capital required to begin construction on a house soon rose to four hundred dollars. On Father de Nisco's recommendation the Bangor banks agreed to lend money for building, allowing ten years for repayment. He attempted to improve the lot of the men in the quarries, who were grossly underpaid and over-worked. After failing in negotiations with the quarry owners, he organized a labor union, appointing himself as president. Shortly thereafter he called a strike, and quarry owners imported a hundred southern blacks as strikebreakers. When the blacks saw the dangerous quarry pits, however, they refused to work and soon returned home. The priest was ultimately successful in increasing workers' wages to $1.50 for a nine-hour day. On another occasion, when a smallpox epidemic erupted in the town, he closed the quarries again by imposing a quarantine on the citizens. In addition, he urged them to become immunized.

To counter a tendency of the men to frequent the bars in Bangor, Father de Nisco recommended that they obtain a wholesale liquor license. He hoped his people would enjoy light wines and beer, to which they were accustomed at home, "under their own vine and fig trees."

Further civic progress was achieved through a series of successful petitions. One to the Postal Service in 1898 achieved a local post office; with it the name New Italy was abandoned and the town was officially named Roseto. Another successful petition, this time to the Northampton County Court, created a separate electoral seat in Washington Township of Roseto so that it would no longer be necessary for Rosetans to travel three miles to vote. After that petition was granted, the Rosetans began taking an interest in local and national politics. In 1920, although most Rosetans were Republican, a Roseto Democratic Club was organized.

A weekly newspaper, *La Stella di Roseto*, established in 1902 in nearby Pen Argyl, provided communication among Italians in Northampton county. It continued publication until its owner's death in 1936. Relationships between Roseto Italians and those living in surrounding towns were further enhanced by the organization in Roseto of the Guglielmo Marconi Pleasure Club in 1903, later known as the Marconi Social Club. The following year, to secure legalization of the club, the members required that the club's officers must be American citizens. A petition for incorporation was granted the club in 1905, after which the building was enlarged and modernized and became a focal point for social activities in the community.[36]

Father de Nisco urged the young girls of the community to become wage earners, encouraging many of them to work in the shirt factory in Bangor. Ultimately preferring to keep all the interests of his people concentrated in their town and in their church, however, the priest appealed to the wealthier residents of Roseto to establish their own shirt factory, and in 1905 the first such factory was built. Soon it was producing seventy dozen shirts a day. Shares in the company sold initially at ten dollars each. The girls operating the machines were paid by piecework, thereby supplementing family income by about six to eight dollars a week. Although the factory was usually shorthanded because the girls one after another would marry and quit work, it was a standby for hard times and boredom.

Immigration from Roseto Val Fortore and some of the neighboring towns continued apace. By 1905, with a population of more than 1,500, and with ninety-six registered voters, Roseto potentially controlled the balance of political power in Washington Township. Nevertheless, its schools had the poorest teachers in the township, and its unpaved and unlighted streets were often impassable. Father de Nisco mobilized the voters and soon obtained a new road. By 1906 Roseto, having realized the power of its votes, prepared to incorporate, although some of the citizens, especially the landowners, feared that incorporation would result in higher taxes. Even Father de Nisco was skeptical that his *paesani* could govern themselves. The first petition for incorporation was rejected by the court.

In the midst of Roseto's growing pains the Archbishop of Philadelphia offered Father de Nisco the pastorate of one of that city's well-established churches, where he would find responsibilities less taxing and a respite from his labors. Declining the offer he replied, "I want to die with my boots on."

A second petition for incorporation succeeded, spurred by the vigorous support of younger Rosetans and persuasive editorials in the newspaper, *La Stella di Roseto*. Thereupon, as Roseto became an independent borough, a special election was held in 1912 to select its officials. Roseto thus became the first American municipality governed by Italians. Father de Nisco, the architect of Roseto, died in 1911 following an appendectomy and so missed by a year the event that gave his town full independent status. Roseto at the time of his death had grown to 328.5 acres with nearly 300 homes and a total assessed value of $175,000.

In the year following incorporation, Columbus Public Grade School was constructed in Roseto, and in 1918 Boy Scout troops were established in the Catholic and Presbyterian churches. The Roseto First National Bank was chartered in 1927, but closed its doors six years later during the depression. By 1930 there were 1,746 Italian Americans in Roseto. A town hall was dedicated in 1935; De Nisco Park and athletic field were incorporated in 1938; the Salesian Sisters Convent and parochial kindergarten were built in 1940; the American Legion Martocci-Capobianco Post No. 750 was organized in 1945; Pius X High School was constructed in 1947. In 1951 the Community Board of Trade (Chamber of Commerce) was formed to better relations between merchants and the Town Council; in 1952 the mayor of Roseto Val Fortore in Italy visited the town; in 1953 Our Lady of Mt. Carmel Elementary School was completed; in 1962 Roseto celebrated its fiftieth year as an incorporated Italian-American community. The antagonism and scorn of its neighbors described in chapter 1 had gradually faded over the years. In fact, a degree of admiration and even jealousy of Roseto's prosperity had emerged as Rosetans began to accede to leadership positions in the larger community of Pennsylvania's slate belt.

3

A Medical Study
of Neighboring Communities
with Contrasting Social Patterns

Having confirmed the remarkably low death rate from myocardial infarction in Roseto observed by Dr. Benjamin Falcone, who, as cited in chapter 1, had practiced medicine in Roseto and Bangor for seventeen years, we felt the need to look for evidences of coronary disease among the living and to compare our findings in Roseto with other communities in the area. One of us (Stewart Wolf) obtained an introduction to the chairman of the Roseto Town Council through a resident of Roseto, a carpenter named Anthony Guida, who was working at Totts Gap at the time. Mr. Guida persuaded his sister-in-law, Lucille Guida, to arrange an interview with her father, Domenico Martino, at his home in Roseto. Dr. Wolf hoped to obtain his permission and his support with the town leaders for an extensive medical survey of the community.

Mr. Martino's daughter, Lucille, answered the doorbell and ushered Dr. Wolf into the living room, where Mr. Martino and his wife sat on a couch. Lucille and her husband, Louis Guida, occupied two of the chairs, and a third, across from Mr. Martino, had been reserved for Dr. Wolf. After a short exchange of pleasantries, Lucille retired to the kitchen, only to appear a few minutes later with wine and food. After another short interval of small talk, Mr. Martino suddenly said, "Well Dr. Wolf, what can we do to help you?" After the purpose of the study, the proposed method, and the number and type of personnel involved had been laid out before him, Mr. Martino promised his support. He suggested a preliminary testing period, which, if it went well, could be followed by a full-scale examination of the inhabitants of the community. He offered the Town Council chambers, located on the upper floor of the firehouse, as a site for the preliminary clinic the first two weeks in December 1962. The visit concluded with Mr. Martino's assurance that he would bring the proposal before the Town Council.

Permission was granted by the mayor and council within two weeks. The mayor, George Giaquinto, then arranged for Dr. Wolf to meet with him and his sister, Florence Giaquinto, at her home on Garibaldi Avenue, where she lived with her severely arthritic sister, Palma, and a niece, Donna. Florence and her sisters, Rose Cistone, Virginia Donatelli, and Mary Carrescia volunteered to act as receptionists and clerks during the examination to record the personal data, including the names and locations of parents, grandparents, and children.

The Setting

Roseto is located in Northampton County, Pennsylvania, once a portion of Bucks County, which, along with Philadelphia and Chester counties, were the three original counties established by William Penn in 1682. Bucks County had extended north to the New York colony, west to the Susquehanna River, and east to the Delaware River. Northampton County was formed from the most northerly and largest section of Bucks. Later, portions of Northampton were carved off to form a dozen other counties, which, along with Northampton County, remain today.

Roseto lies beneath the Appalachian Ridge, where it forms the northern border of Northampton County (fig. 3.1). There, at 1,600 feet above sea level, it extends east and west from the Delaware Water Gap to the gap through which the Lehigh River flows. The geological character of the county has allowed for the establishment of several industries. Immediately below the ridge, under flat-topped hills and small valleys that range from 600 to 900 feet above sea level, lies a ribbon of slate and shale six to nine miles wide. Roseto is located near the eastern end of this slate belt where most of the early Rosetans were employed.

FIGURE 3.1

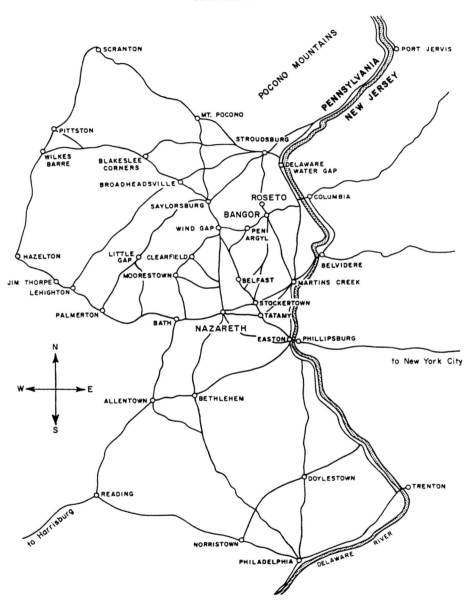

Roseto and Environs

The Industrial Environment

The first slate quarry was opened in Bushkill Township in 1812, but not until the early 1860s did the slate industry become established. It was developed by Welsh immigrants from Bangor and vicinity in North Wales, a major center for slate production. Familiar with the methods of finding, quarrying, and shaping slate, the Welsh immigrants settled in the richest veins and established communities that they named after their home towns of Pen Argyl and Bangor in Wales.

South of the slate belt stretching east to the approximate longitude of the Wind Gap, the terrain, 400 to 450 feet above sea level, is much flatter. Here, beneath the surface, is a band of limestone about seven miles wide, the raw material for the cement industry. Here, too, the land was ideal for farming

In the southern portion of Northampton County, between Easton and Bethlehem, lies a belt of iron ore that was mined before 1800 by several small mining companies. Following the depression of 1873, most of them merged to form the Bethlehem Iron Company, which eventually became Bethlehem Steel. The success of steel making depended heavily on the development of the Bessemer method of removing part of the carbon from molten iron. Readily accessible anthracite coal was also important to the steel industry, and abundant coal was discovered in 1790 in what is now known as Carbon County, but which was then part of Northampton County.

Another early industry, inaugurated in 1770, was lumber. Farming, however, was the major occupation of the inhabitants of mainly rural Northampton County. Small dairy farms of 90 to 300 acres were scattered throughout the county. Most of them are still active, and some belong to descendants of the original settlers who arrived in the region as early as 1720.

Before the Penn family could establish ownership through occupation of the entire area, Northampton County was already populated by French traders and Scottish immigrants from northern Ireland, most of whom were escaping political oppression and economic privation during the early reign of King William III of England. By 1740 members of the Protestant Moravian sect from southern Germany had settled Nazareth and then Bethlehem; Dutch Protestants and French Huguenots had also migrated into the northern portion of the county from New York. Soon new waves of impecunious Germans and Irish were arriving through Philadelphia by the mechanism of the "redemptioner," whereby shipmasters would provide free passage to migrants if they agreed to be sold for three to five years into indentured service before regaining their freedom. The various ethnic groups, chiefly farmers and traders, remained more or less segregated in small towns scattered throughout the county. Italian immigrants did not begin arriving in large numbers until the latter two decades of the nineteenth century (table 3.1).

The Rosetans became part of the flood of Italian immigrants during the 1880s. They settled in a rough terrain where the road rises sharply at the northern edge of the Bangor business district along Martins Creek. Viewed from the east, Roseto appears terraced, with homes nestled on the slopes. The highest and lowest elevations are, respectively, 720 feet and 620 feet above sea level. Its streets are coextensive with those of Bangor.

TABLE 3.1
The Italian Emigration to America by Decades
According to Historical Statistics of the United States

1821–1830	409
1831–1840	2.,253
1841–1850	1,870
1851–1860	9,231
1861–1870	11,725
1871–1880	55,759
1881–1890	307,309
1891–1900	651,893
1901–1910	2,045,877
1911–1920	1,109,524
1921–1930	455,315
1931–1940	68,028

The present town covers a land area of one-half square mile. Narrow cement streets, many bearing Italian names, are now pretty well covered

with asphalt. The main street, Garibaldi Avenue, connects the northern
and southern boundaries of the town. Our first impression of Roseto in
1962 was of an extremely clean, neat, well-kept town. The streets were
named after Italian heroes, Columbus, Dante, and Garibaldi, American
presidents or the earliest settlers of Roseto. They were lined with red
brick and varicolored frame houses almost abutting the sidewalk. Most
had front porches where the families sat, especially on weekends, watch-
ing activities on the street or talking with neighbors or passersby. There
were only a few feet between houses, but behind each one was a lawn
and garden extending the width of the house and thirty yards or more to
the rear. Although there were a few flowers, the gardens contained mainly
vegetables and grape arbors.

The 350 houses in the town were mainly two-story frame dwellings
with three generations of one family occupying most of them. Others,
divided into apartments, were occupied by two or three families of one
clan. The dwellings along Garibaldi Avenue and adjacent streets also
contained Roseto's more than forty small businesses. Two Italian baker-
ies operated by a pair of cousins were located in the basements of the
homes. Bread, pizza, fish pie, pasta, and pretzels were baked daily. There
was also a meat market. The five restaurants in the town and three
adjoining bars all occupied the first floors of their owners' residences.
Sixteen textile factories scattered throughout the town constituted the
remaining local industry. Altogether, in Roseto and the immediately
adjacent areas, there were thirty of these factories.

Roseto's population remained fairly stable after its first census in
1920, until a gradual decline in population began in 1950 (table 3.2) and
a sharp decline in the birth rate began in 1967 (table 3.3). During the first
half of the twentieth century most Rosetan families had six or more
children, but by 1950 the number had dwindled. Most couples had one
to three children, and 12 percent were childless. Most young Rosetan
couples lived with parents or other family members, and more than half
of the single, widowed, or divorced persons lived with family members.
Infants were breast-fed by their mothers but were mothered by many
females in the family including older sisters, aunts, grandmothers, and
even cousins. As they grew up, the children played mainly with their own
relatives and nearby neighbors.

TABLE 3.2
Population of Roseto, 1920–1970

Year	Total Population
1920	1,643
1930	1,746
1940	1,778
1950	1,676
1960	1,630
1970	1,538
1980	1,484
1990	1,555

Source: U.S. Census of Population. No census data are available for 1910, since Roseto was not incorporated as a borough until 1912.

TABLE 3.3
Number of Resident Live Births and Total Deaths
for Roseto, Bangor, and Nazareth, 1961–1971
(Rate per 1,000 Estimated Mid-year Population

	ROSETO				BANGOR				NAZARETH			
Year	Number of Births	Rate	Number of Deaths	Rate	Number of Births	Rate	Number of Deaths	Rate	Number of Births	Rate	Number of Deaths	Rate
1961	21	12.9	11	6.7	81	14.1	64	11.1	95	15.3	71	11.5
1962	27	16.7	14	8.6	96	16.8	67	11.7	124	20.2	86	14.0
1963	19	11.8	13	8.0	84	14.8	63	11.1	121	19.8	87	14.2
1964	22	13.7	13	8.0	114	20.2	100	17.7	130	21.4	88	14.5
1965	26	16.3	18	11.3	83	14.7	77	13.7	103	17.0	90	14.9
1966	34	21.4	22	13.9	85	15.2	81	14.5	104	17.3	81	13.5
1967	11	6.9	22	13.9	72	12.9	67	12.0	100	16.7	101	16.9
1968	17	10.8	11	7.0	68	12.3	87	15.7	107	18.0	75	12.6
1969	20	12.8	15	9.6	85	15.4	65	11.8	94	15.9	77	13.0
1970	11	7.0	13	8.3	71	13.0	74	13.5	104	17.7	66	11.2
1971	17	11.0	16	10.3	62	11.4	77	14.1	81	13.9	91	15.6

Source: Department of Health, Commonwealth of Pennsylvania, Harrisburg.

At the time of our initial study, a few older Rosetans still made their own wine, half of which they gave away to friends and relatives. They made one batch in November from imported California Concord grapes, and a second wine from grapes they grew in the backyards of their homes. Their gardens were also planted with Italian lettuce, cabbage, green peppers, onions, peas, beans, endives, radishes, eggplant, tomatoes, corn, beets, cucumbers, figs, peaches, pears, apples, pumpkins, cherries, plums, parsley, oregano, mint, and various other spices. The Rosetans canned much of their produce for the winter.

In the early 1960s most adult Rosetans were second- or third-genera-tion Italians. The 18 percent of Rosetans married to non-Italians (English, Welsh, Pennsylvania Dutch) still suffered mild social disapproval. In contrast to most American communities, life expectancy for men in Roseto was slightly longer than that for women. Indeed, we found a few more widowers than widows in the town, although over all, females outnumbered males five to four. Table 3.4 records the life expectancies of all age groups 21 years and older. Table 3.5 defines marital status.

Traditional Beliefs and Behavior

As described by Clement Valletta, a young social scientist born near Roseto, the community evolved from the well-defined culture of south-ern Italian peasants, *contadini*.[32] Most had retained a centuries-old belief in, and fear of, supernatural forces usually set in motion by strong desires, or *voli*.[33] Supernatural beliefs were closely intertwined with deep, reli-gious Christian faith and dependence on the good will of the Virgin Mary. Unfavorable circumstances attributable to *malocchio*, the evil eye, were thought to be brought on by envious, evil, or vindictive *voli* of others. Natural disasters such as storms, floods, and droughts were accepted as matters of fate, sometimes inflicted because of intense human desires (*voli*). According to Valletta: "When times were hard the villager knew it was useless to argue with fate. With almost a Greek sense of destiny, Rosetans accepted the inevitable even while they prayed for Divine intercession. They felt as much at home in their universe as did medieval men who saw their firmament alive with symbols of good and evil, right and wrong."[32]

TABLE 3.4
Percentage Distribution of Rosetans over Age 24 by Sex and Age in 1960

Age	Males N = %		Females N = %		Totals N = %	
25–34	109	14	118	14	227	14
35–44	121	16	143	17	264	16
45–54	102	13	145	17	247	15
55–64	69	9	63	7	132	8
65 & over	71	9	75	9	146	9
Totals	472	61%	544	64%	898	62%

TABLE 3.5
Marital Status in Roseto

Men and Women	N = %	
Married once *	663	74
Married more than once	18	2
Separated or divorced	33	4
Widowed (more men than women)	70	8
Single (more women than men)	124	14

Further demographic data on the population of Roseto revealed that the mean age at marriage for men was 24.6, and the mean age for women was 22.1 years.

The fatalistic attitude of the Rosetans also marked their acceptance of the death of a child or young person despite its being accompanied by deep feelings of sorrow. The death of a spouse was similarly experienced but the grief was more palpable. A startling number of surviving spouses died within a year or two or even within days, weeks, or months of their deceased mate. The attitude toward the death of an older parent resembled that toward a harvest: the culmination of a natural cycle of planting the seed, cultivation, maturity, and death, followed by fresh new growth. Young children sometimes attended funerals. The collation that followed was a warm, friendly, almost cheerful celebration of the loved one who had left the fold for a heavenly reward.

Social Structure

Valletta noted that after nearly one hundred years of exposure to American traditions, Rosetans still clung to their hierarchical family structure and felt the need to protect themselves against community malediction by admonishing their children to avoid offending others.[32]

Those who were descended from, or were otherwise related to, the original settlers held the highest social position. Their extended families tended to become the nuclei of fairly well defined clans. A bride usually joined the clan of her husband, unless her clan had a higher social position by virtue of its connection to the early days of Roseto, in which case her husband and children were usually assumed into her own clan.

Most clans had an identifiable patriarch and matriarch, the respected elders. The active leader, or "prime minister" of the clan, might be the owner of the blouse mill or another well-to-do man in the age group 45 to 65. His cabinet of advisers was usually made up of brothers and sisters, at least one of whom had some advanced education. In matters requiring serious consideration or action, the patriarch acted as the "supreme court." Despite its clearly organized structure, family life was relaxed and informal. Backyard celebrations marked every important event: birthdays, anniversaries, religious holidays, first communion, high school graduation, engagement, or marriage. Family and friends gathered in the spacious backyard of one of the houses for a feast prepared and served by the women. The men circulated with pitchers of red wine poured over peaches, while the guests helped themselves to sausages, pizzas, and a variety of Italian delicacies.

Social Life and Institutions

The social life of Roseto revolved around its twenty-two social and civic organizations, the largest of which were the American Legion, the Rod and Gun Club, the Marconi Social Club, the Columbia Fire Company, and the Holy Name Society. Most of these organizations were for men, although some of them had women's auxiliaries. Otherwise, the women were excluded from the clubs except on special occasions. Activities in the clubs consisted of bantering, bragging, joking, and Italian drinking games (*morra*) and card games (*briscola* and *tresette*). Men in the fire company cooked occasional meals in their club kitchen.

Of the Rosetan men whom we canvassed, 81 percent were members of at least one community organization. Of those who were members 94 percent were apparently active members. Sixty-three percent of the respondents (mainly those over 30) had expressed the opinion that it was necessary to be active in organizations if one lived in Roseto. Rosetans aged 21 to 30, most of whom were not affiliated with organizations, felt that such membership was not important. Those active in the Marconi Club, the first social organization in the community, were mainly 65 and over; those in the age group 55 to 64 made up most of the membership of the fire company; while those aged 31 to 44 belonged mainly to the Knights of Columbus. Such community organizations, as they bridged the gap between family activities and solitude, were powerful contributors to Roseto's close-knit character.

The social life of Rosetan women revolved around their work in the blouse mills and their participation in church groups, the parent-teachers association, and women's auxiliary groups, as well as from the joint preparation of meals for special family and religious occasions.

The teenagers' gathering place was Mary's Luncheonette, where their behavior for the most part was quiet and restrained. Mary Bert, as they called her, served an important function as impresario and facilitator of the social life of young people. She would know which boy a young girl was interested in and vice versa, so if one of them came into the little restaurant, she would phone to inform the other one that circumstances were favorable.

During the day the community was quiet and appeared deserted because nearly all adult Rosetans of both sexes and all ages had jobs. In the evening the men gathered at their social clubs and the women in their homes.

Otherwise, in the evening when the weather permitted, most Rosetans walked around the town, stopping from time to time to chat with neighbors, to compare notes, or to argue vigorously over some political issue. The town was then exclusively Italian except for three or four families; one of Greek origin and another, Latin American, had adopted the Italian pattern of living and, except for their names, were clearly identified by their neighbors as Rosetans.

Disturbances in the town were rare and there was virtually no petty crime. Thus the local police were called upon mainly to direct traffic for funerals and at the annual festival of Our Lady of Mt. Carmel. Roseto's volunteer fire department was an important social institution. With only a rare small blaze to fight, the men engaged in frequent drills to keep their newly acquired modern fire truck in working order. The second floor of the fire house was a men's club and bar open to the volunteer firemen and friends who contributed financially. The third and top floor was the headquarters of the Town Council.

The Roseto Story 1962–1963

The preliminary survey took place in the Town Council chamber during the first two weeks of December 1962. The necessary arrangements had been made by Florence Giaquinto, her sisters, and a few other women by the time the Oklahoma team of physicians, dieticians, and laboratory technicians appeared to begin work. Places for each type of examination and testing were sectioned off into compartments around the edges of the large Council Hall surrounding a central reception desk. At the entrance there were chairs for the waiting patients. Rosetan men and women poured in throughout the day. Since many selected the lunch hour or the period just before or after, the Oklahoma staff worked without interruption from 9:00 A.M. to 6:00 P.M. Sandwiches for the workers were provided by midday everyday, however, by various women of the community. Their hospitality extended to the dinner hour as well, and many members of the group were invited to their homes. The remainder usually ate together at one of several small restaurants in Roseto.

During the short two weeks of the preliminary survey, the Council chamber took on the air of a social gathering place; the atmosphere was cheerful and neighborly, with much good-natured kidding and joking. Most of the patients expressed appreciation of the thorough medical survey evaluation offered to them without cost. In each case, if requested, the findings were communicated to their physicians, who, for their part, encouraged their patients to attend the clinic. The Oklahomans were impressed by the friendly, optimistic atmosphere of Roseto, the hospitality, the relaxed but very dignified and almost courtly behavior of the citizens, their close family ties, and especially their lack of ostentation.

The preliminary medical survey having gone well, the major part of the study was undertaken the following summer (1963). A larger contingent of physicians, dieticians, sociologists, and technicians participated from June through August, this time working in the Columbus School building. Again, the townspeople were hospitable and helpful. The same volunteers plus a few others helped with managing the entire procedure. The main study hall served as the reception area and the surrounding classrooms and a few curtained-off areas were used for the individual parts of the survey: medical history; physical examination; dietary, smoking, and drinking inquiry; sociological interview; and electrocardiogram and blood tests. The methods and procedures used are described in chapter 4.

A Similar Investigation in Bangor

The summer of 1964 was devoted to the study of the inhabitants of Bangor, a town immediately adjacent to Roseto, which was served by the same water company, the same physicians, and the same regional hospitals. Again, local volunteers helped with the arrangements and the conduct of the survey. From the observations of the investigators, the behavior of the Bangorians differed sharply from that of the Rosetans. They interacted much less with each other during the clinic sessions, were less jovial and more restrained, and, by dress, speech, and general demeanor, class differences were much more evident among them. While most Bangorians were appreciative of the free examination, they appeared to be enjoying the survey less than did the Rosetans.

From documentation described in chapter 8, Bangor's social structure was far less cohesive than that of Roseto. The community had never been altogether ethnically or socially homogeneous. When the Welsh established the slate industry in the area during the 1860s, they incorporated a cluster of four small villages; Howell-Town, Cricktown, Newvillage and Uttsville. All had been established a century before by the original settlers, Scotch-Irish and German Mennonite farmers.

As Bangor's slate industry grew and prospered, other businesses were established; glove manufacturing plants, a large silk company, foundries, and mills. Bangor remained economically healthy until the depression of the early 1930s. When the economy recovered, the slate industry prospered again for a few years until the Johns Manville Company's development of asbestos roofing shingles delivered the coup de grâce to slate as a preferred roofing material, setting off serious rivalry among the several ethnic groups.

Italians comprised nearly 25 percent of the Bangor population in 1960. Two-thirds of them were members of Roseto families, and two-thirds of those lived in the Fourth ward of Bangor, which adjoined Roseto at the site of Our Lady of Mt. Carmel Church and close to the most densely populated part of Roseto. A large number of Poles comprised the other mainly Catholic portion of the population. There were eight Protestant churches in Bangor, Methodist, Presbyterian, Lutheran, Dutch Reform, and Moravian but only a single Roman Catholic church, although a third of Bangor's population of more than 5,000 were Roman Catholic. Consequently, many of the Italians worshipped at Our Lady of Mt. Carmel in adjacent Roseto.

As noted earlier, the lack of social cohesion in Bangor stood in sharp contrast to the tightly knit social structure of Roseto. One of the protestant ministers told us: "We have no membership directory. There is a looseness in the organization of the church and an 'I don't care' attitude about neighbors." Another minister said that only half the members of his church attended regularly. "We don't have involvement," he said. "They don't want to get involved even on Sunday mornings, but they resent it very much if they are told that their membership has lapsed, because when they die they want it to be known that they belonged to a church." He and the other Protestant clergymen spoke longingly of the sense of commitment of parishioners in Roseto.

The lack of community cohesion and individual loyalty to the community of Bangor was also evident in the economic and political spheres. There were nearly fifty families whose assets were estimated at $100,000 or more. For the most part they declined to involve themselves in community projects and politics. The mayor's efforts to launch a committee of citizens to "uplift" the town was frustrated on the one hand by indifference, and on the other by ethnic antagonisms. Many townspeople expressed disdain for neighbors who had become successful in business or had gained any social prominence.

Nazareth

During the third summer, the team from Oklahoma examined the inhabitants of Nazareth, a town located about ten miles from Roseto, which had been settled in 1740 by Moravians, a southern German religious group.

For more than a hundred years, only members of the Moravian church were allowed to live in Nazareth. In 1850 the ban was lifted because of economic necessity. Nazareth soon became a "prestige address" for immigrants with Germanic ethnic connections, especially for those who left Germany during the 1848 revolution, for Austro-Hungarians who escaped military service during World War I, and for those who emigrated after the war. These immigrants added several Lutheran churches to the two original Moravian churches. During the late nineteenth century and early twentieth century, the growing cement and steel industries attracted many Italian and central and eastern European Roman Catholic immigrants to the prosperous, attractive town of Nazareth.

Once a rigidly regulated enclave of religiously devoted Bohemians and Moravians, Nazareth became a prosperous, socially and ethnically diverse, fairly typical small American city. We found that the Nazarenes were more sophisticated and more prosperous than Bangorians and Rosetans. Among them the Moravians occupied a higher social status than the less cultivated "Pennsylvania Dutch," who outnumbered them but who spoke "impure" German. At the time of our study 70 percent of the population were Protestant and 20 percent Roman Catholic. A few families adhered to small fundamentalist Protestant groups.

Post War Social Flux

All three towns, Roseto, Bangor, and Nazareth had been undergoing social change, especially since World War II. The horizons of many young Rosetans were widened during their military service. Moreover, the cohesive forces of the war and the subsequent comparative prosperity brought Rosetans in the region into closer contact and cooperation with people in neighboring communities.

As the Rosetans became more educated, more prosperous, and more sophisticated, traditional patterns of living began to erode somewhat, although at the time of our initial study, close family and community ties were still strikingly evident in Roseto. We visited 86 percent of households in Roseto in 1966. The information gathered reflected the persistence of family solidarity (table 3.6).

The Young People (Bangor and Roseto)

We conducted several interviews with groups of teenagers in Roseto and Bangor in 1963. The boys and girls were asked questions regarding their attitudes toward their towns, their educational aspirations, and their involvement in school and community activities. Roseto teenagers expressed a greater degree of attachment to family than did Bangor Italian and non-Italian teenagers. Both Roseto and Bangor Italian teenagers, however, belonged to fewer organized peer groups than did the Bangor non-Italians. Thus, Italian youth in general were primarily "homebound," associating with peers of their own ethnic group rather than joining school or community organizations.

TABLE 3.6
Distribution of the Population of Roseto on the
Family Solidarity Index, 1966 (N = 898)

	N = %	
1. Subject is living with spouse	663	74
2. Subject is of the same ethnicity as spouse	663	74
3. Subject is of the same religion as spouse	690	70
4. Subject has lived in Roseto entire life	490	55
5. Spouse has lived in Roseto entire life	380	42
6. Three-generation households	620	69
7. Subject and spouse spend time with other people	175	19
8. All children live at home	560	62
9. Children are married to Italians	520	58
10. Subject turns to family with problems	632	70
11. All siblings live in Roseto	150	17
12. Subject attends family reunions	304	34

There was very little evidence of adolescent rebellion among Roseto teenagers. For the most part they were tractable and well behaved but were nevertheless restless and expressed dissatisfaction with opportunities in Roseto. Rejecting the prevailing mores in Roseto, they aspired to live as middle-class Americans.

Most of the adolescents expressed a need for independence from the restricted life of Roseto. Nevertheless, they were uncertain as to the likelihood of success of their independent efforts and the degree of satisfaction that middle-class rewards might provide.

Still under the influence of Father de Nisco's teaching, parents in Roseto had sacrificed to provide education for their children, even to the level of college and professional school. They took pride in the fact that more than 150 of them had entered semiprofessional or professional occupations since the turn of the century.

Few of the older generation had had much schooling, but those between the ages of 30 and 45 had, for the most part, achieved a high school education. Despite the ready availability of public education, most Rosetan children still attended the parochial elementary and high schools, and 80 percent of the high school graduates attended college. Only 2 percent of the population, however, had gone on to graduate or professional schools. The Rosetan teenagers found that after specialized training, they did not fit into the Rosetan culture. To quote one of them:

There is very little excitement, no industry, which is the reason for young college graduates to abandon this town. There is no place to get ahead. Other than the mills, there is nothing a person can do for a living. The children in Roseto have a chance for a good education, but it is hard to live in Roseto if you acquire a specialized education. All Rosetans have a higher goal, but the old people want to keep things the way they are used to.

Yet some Rosetan teenagers seemed ambivalent about compromising their way of life, and some voiced concern for the future of their town. The comments of three such Rosetan teenagers went essentially as follows:

I think Roseto is a fairly good town in which to live. There is a deep security in knowing when problems are to be faced. Most people in town can rely on certain members of the family to help them solve these problems. There are many opportunities for children to develop socially because of the closeness or affinity people have for one another. The town also faces serious problems. Some of these are related to the lack of sufficient job opportunities for men. Because of the lack of well-paying job opportunities, women must work and men must usually leave the town to find better jobs. I think that this problem leaves much to be desired in the cultural development and broad-mindedness of most of the people in the town. Most of the people are well off financially, but they must work too hard for what they have. I think the people are very happy in the town. They have a firm belief in God and desire better conditions for their children.

I think Roseto is a very good place in which to live, but I do not think I will live here after my education is completed. I say this because I do not expect to find a job in this area. However, I feel I have gained much by growing up in Roseto, and I would like to live in a town similar to it in size and location. Knowing many of the people in the town definitely has its faults, but it also has its advantages, which I feel outweigh the former. I am proud of my Italian heritage and the fact that many Rosetans are now very successful, although they had little to start with.

I feel safe and completely happy being in Roseto; for some strange reason I do not want to leave Roseto. It is peaceful. There are no gangs; one is brought up wholesome. The people are sociable. The fact that most of the residents are Italian provides a unified community.

Local Industry and Occupations

Slate mining, initially the principal industry of Roseto and Bangor, had, as mentioned earlier, begun to decline in the 1930s. Further decline occurred as the workers demanded higher and higher wages to work in the hazardous quarry pits, thus increasing the market price for slate and decreasing the demand. Nevertheless, when we studied the community in the early 1960s most of the quarries were still active. Their number in the area diminished, however, from sixteen to half a dozen by the 1970s. Thus many Rosetans were forced to find jobs outside the community in cement and steel mills, in other nearby industries, or in road construction as skilled laborers. A few were salesmen, technicians, or proprietors of their own small businesses in or near Roseto.

The economy of Roseto was dependent primarily on sixteen small textile factories that finished women's blouses and one paper-box factory. Nearly three-quarters of the women in Roseto worked in these jointly owned family enterprises. Most of the lawyers, engineers, physicians, dentists, osteopaths, and chiropractors who grew up in Roseto lived in Bangor or other nearby towns. Many of the third-generation, college-educated youth had moved to other parts of the country seeking white-collar jobs. The occupations of Rosetans in 1966 are shown in table 3.7.

Although 87 percent of all Rosetans had achieved more education than their fathers, only 57 percent were employed at higher occupational levels than those of their fathers; 29 percent were at the same occupational level as their fathers; and 14 percent were at a lower level. Those Rosetans who showed the greatest mobility upward and downward were primarily under age 44, while most who were occupationally stable were 65 years old and over.

Twelve percent of the men and 4 percent of the women worked at more than one job, while 25 percent of the men and 4 percent of the women worked more than fifty hours a week in their job. The overall mean annual gross income for employed males and females in 1966 was $6,300 and $2,450, respectively. The combined family incomes of most Rosetan families enabled them to enjoy many middle-class benefits.

TABLE 3.7
Distribution of Rosetans by Sex and Occupation

Occupational Levels *	Males N = %		Females N = %		Totals N = %	
Executives; professionals	5	1	0	0	5	.05
Proprietors of medium-sized business	19	5	14	3	33	4
Administrative personnel; small, independent business owners	47	18	18	4	65	10
Clerical and sales workers; technicians	32	8	27	5	59	7
Skilled manual employees	106	26	8	2	114	13
Machine operators; semiskilled employees	111	28	309	62	420	47
Unskilled employees	53	13	4	0.8	57	6
Housewives	0	0	115	23	115	13
Students	3	0.7	0	0	3	0.3
Total	403		495		898	

* Hollingshead's occupational levels were used.

The Churches

The church of Our Lady of Mt. Carmel, the largest building in Roseto, with a membership of nearly 2,000, straddles the boundary line between Roseto and Bangor. Rosetan parishioners are supplemented by a large number of Italians, mainly relatives of Rosetans living in the Fourth Ward or other parts of Bangor. A small cemetery with elaborate gravestones and monuments lies behind the church. The Presbyterian church, with about 250 members, is a frame structure with an adjoining manse. It stands in the center of town on Garibaldi Avenue. The church of the Jehovah's Witnesses, Kingdom Hall, is just beyond the western edge of town. Nearby, but outside the city limits of Roseto, are two predominantly Italian Episcopal churches. Although there was conflict between Protestants and Catholics in the early days, after Father de Nisco had threatened with excommunication the Rosetans who failed to return to the catholic church, by 1960 there was no social barrier and interdenominational marriages were common.

The Festival of Our Lady of Mt. Carmel

As mentioned in chapter 1 the festival of Our Lady of Mt. Carmel, long a tradition in Roseto Val Fortore was established in Roseto, Pennsylvania, by the early settlers. Although about 16 percent of the Roseto population had maintained their allegiance to the Presbyterian church, and other Protestant denominations were represented as well, the Roman Catholic festival was a celebration for the entire community.

The occasion took place each year during the last week in July. It was preceded by a Wednesday mass, other ceremonies, and a Saturday night carnival. After the Sunday mass the festival queen was crowned. The statue of the Madonna was brought out of the church and placed on a decorated trailer. The selection of the queen was a simple and straightforward matter: She was the senior at Pope Pius School who, among the girls, had shown the most initiative in preparing for the festival. Accompanied by the officers of the Knights of Columbus, she rode with the statue of the Blessed Virgin and the Christ Child, with her court walking behind. A monsignor, born in Roseto, rode in an open Cadillac. The procession moved down the entire length of Garibaldi Avenue a distance of nearly two miles, and back to the church. The music was supplied by the Roseto Cornet Band. The men's and women's religious societies, the Mutual Aid Society of Saint Philip Neri and the Sacred Heart Sodality, marched separately, and the faithful fell in behind. Some of the older women marched barefoot to show humility and their gratitude for the good fortune that had befallen the Rosetans in America.

Administration and Politics

Since its legal recognition as an independent borough in 1912, Roseto had functioned under a burgess or mayor-council form of government. Among the voters, Democrats and Republicans are almost equally represented, but family and clan associations and rivalries are more important than party affiliation in town politics. The mayor, therefore, as a political figurehead, represents his family in directing the town's activities, and thus his successes and failures reflect upon his extended family. Since most Rosetans are Roman Catholic, the priest plays a significant, if informal, role in community politics, chiefly as a personal adviser to the mayor.

Social Values

By 1962 it was evident that beyond its early emphasis on education Roseto now placed a high value on economic success and other competitive activities such as success in charitable drives. With a strong tradition of helping friends as well as family, in Roseto the success of one who has been helped by a friend reflects favorably on the helper.

Luigi Barzini, who emphasized social interdependence as typical of Italians in general, cited as exceptions medicine, law, and other professions that involve a high level of individual responsibility.[23] From the individual interviews conducted during the survey, we learned that although they continued to maintain close family ties, most Rosetans who had achieved professional status rejected Roseto community life and did not return from training to live and practice in the community but transferred to settle in adjacent Bangor or elsewhere. Nevertheless, the people of Roseto were proud of their professionals and often boasted that children from their community had "made good."

The intricate relationship that developed between the town and some of its progeny who had "made good" was described by a successful dentist in Bangor who had been born in Roseto and lived there until he went away to college and dental school. Upon graduation he established an office in Bangor but visited Roseto every Friday to eat spaghetti with his father. "I came from a poor family; my father had a small store in Roseto. I saw my father and brother sacrificing for my education. I couldn't let them down. I owed it to them. A boy has to prove himself to be a champion all the way." He married a Protestant girl of German ancestry, "I wouldn't marry an Italian girl," he explained. "Italian mothers are too possessive of their children; you never know when they're yours or theirs." He said that he and his wife lived mainly to themselves. Most of their friends were of Welsh extraction. He added:

> I feel accepted in Bangor. We're not as excitable or impulsive as Rosetans. People in Roseto are frugal, economical, but for something that shows, they pay a high price. Some people in Roseto embarrass me; they don't know how to reach out, they're still in a shell; they are jealous, belligerent. In Roseto they help you when you're down. When you're up, they cut you down, they throw stones. If you can withstand it, you're a giant, if you crumble, they have no use for you.

By the early 1960s, in the face of obvious impending social change, an unwritten but clear-cut code of proper behavior had evolved for those Rosetans who had achieved material wealth or occupational prestige. The local priest described the required behavioral restraints, which included a delicate balance between ostentation and reserve, personal ambition and concern for others, pride and modesty, lightheartedness and gravity. He emphasized that when preoccupation with earning money exceeded the unmarked boundary, it became a basis for social rejection, irrespective of the standing outside the community. Similarly, a lack of concern for community needs, especially by those who spent their money on frivolous pleasures, constituted grounds for social exclusion.

Rosetan culture thus provided a set of checks and balances to ensure that neither success nor failure got out of hand. Ambition and enhancing one's status were highly valued and expected of the Rosetan male, but overambition was discouraged. Those who had achieved what was regarded as too much power were feared and resented. Those who appeared on the way to prominence were usually required to stand a test of worthiness consisting of verbal affronts by friends and neighbors, the "stone-throwing" referred to earlier. The community, having supported a person in the achievement of his goal, tested his ability to carry success with appropriate grace, humility, and loyalty to his people. The testing ordeal resembled *the dozens*, a term derived from a Scottish word meaning to stun and widely practiced by black groups in which the members of the group, after choosing a leader, revile and insult him for several minutes to test his equanimity, resilience, and good humor.

Social Stratification

During our first study in 1962-63 it was difficult to distinguish, on the basis of dress or behavior, the wealthy from the impecunious in Roseto. Living arrangements (houses and cars) were simple and strikingly similar. Despite the affluence of many, there was at that time no atmosphere of "keeping up with the Joneses" in Roseto, no "putting on the dog." In most families both husbands and wives worked, and virtually all the women did their own housework. As already noted, poorer families were quietly provided for, usually by their relatives.

Social distinctions depended more on family than income. Although descendants of the original settlers from Roseto Val Fortore enjoyed especially high status, it could also be earned by working hard for the community, living by the rules, and upholding community standards, or by attaining a college or professional education. Solid, dependable citizenship, home ownership and meticulous maintenance of one's home, regular attendance at church, generous subscription to charitable and other community causes were the marks of those accorded the greatest respect. Italian Americans who were not Roseto natives were well accepted in the community, but only conditionally until they had learned the English language and demonstrated conformity to local customs and values.

Gans described four major behavior types among Italian Americans in Boston's West End, which we found applied to some extent in Roseto.[37] He distinguished routine seekers, middle-class mobiles, action seekers, and maladapted. The routine seekers in Roseto were mainly first-and second-generation families who held firmly to Old World traditions and lived by established patterns. They found security and satisfaction in familiar and predictable circumstances. Even the food items to be eaten on certain days of the week were clearly prescribed and adhered to. Somewhat younger and, at the time our study began, in much smaller numbers were the middle-class mobiles, who sought "social advancement" in professional education and business contacts outside Roseto. A few of these, especially the more affluent, became action seekers as reflected in their inclinations toward entertainment and travel and in their more mercenary attitudes. The maladapted, initially very few, were mainly those who had broken away from Rosetan traditions by marrying non-Italians, by spending money freely, or by dissociating themselves from formerly close family and community ties. The balance appeared to us to be shifting toward a larger proportion of middle-class mobiles and action seekers. Indeed, the interviews conducted in 1963 with individuals below 35 years of age, some of whom were born during the Great Depression of 1929 to 1934, together with our interviews with teenagers, led us confidently to predict impending social change as early as 1963.

4

Strategy of Inquiry: Subjects, Methods, and Hypothesis Testing

Firm evidence attesting to the significance of psychosocial factors in coronary artery disease has been tantalizingly elusive. Most published studies have focused on fragments of the social experience such as observable behavioral characteristics (Type A),[8] ways of interpreting challenges and stresses (Sisyphus),[38] specific stresses (economic or educational handicap),[39] emotional tendencies (hostility).[40] Those that have dealt with social correlates of health and longevity have been concerned mainly with ethnic, occupational, or demographic groupings, although there have been important studies of social support as a protection against heart attack.[41]

Groen, one of the early workers in the field of psychosocial factors in coronary disease, urged, as a more comprehensive approach, the study of a constellation of pathogenic and protective factors including (a) an identified stressful circumstance or environment, (b) an individual's proclivity for responding to challenge, (c) his or her coping style, and (d) available social and emotional resources.[42]

The recognition of the impact of social pressures on the behavior of the heart and coronary arteries has been implicit in colloquial language for centuries in such expressions as "a broken heart," "a heavy heart," "my heart stood still," "heart throb," and so forth. Physicians in practice, von Dusch in 1868[43] and later Osler[44] in his 1910 Lumelian lecture, have identified social struggle as pertinent to the manifestations of coronary heart disease.

Circumstances unfolding in Roseto over the past twenty-five years have afforded an opportunity to study prospectively, on the one hand, the significance of social support to health and longevity and, on the other, the relevance of the stressful accompaniments of rapid social change to coronary heart disease.

As mentioned in the previous chapter, Old World values and behaviors, marked by family solidarity and community cohesion, were still prominent among Roseto's inhabitants when we began to study the town in 1962. Many of the early immigrants were still alive, as were their children born during the first few years after immigration. The Rosetans of later generations, however, remote as they were from the early years of hardship and ethnic discrimination, expressed little interest in traditional social values and, instead, aspired to the more materialistic satisfactions urged on them by radio and television commercials and enjoyed by their neighbors. Barzini had noted comparable changes among Italians in Italy. Writing in the 1960s, he observed; "also in Italy modern life is eroding the splendid solidity of the family. The change could clearly have serious consequences."[23] As the young Rosetans in Pennsylvania grew to assume leadership in the community, and as many of the older citizens died off, a rapid and radical social change began and became clearly evident by the mid 1960s.

The Continuing Study of Roseto

In early 1962 death certificates covering the years 1955 through 1961 from Roseto and four control communities within a ten mile radius of Roseto, Bangor, Nazareth, Stroudsburg, and East Stroudsburg, were obtained from the Division of Vital Statistics of the Department of Health of the Commonwealth of Pennsylvania.

To verify the data on death certificates, the clinical records of each individual whose cause of death had been judged to be due to a cardiovascular or pulmonary disorder were searched for in the six regional hospitals that served the inhabitants of the five communities. Hospital records of 75 percent of the deceased were located and studied to verify the cause of death as recorded on the death certificates.[45] Additional information on each subject was obtained from the practicing physicians who served the five communities. The mortality records, verified insofar as possible, were then classified according to cause of death: myocardial infarction or sudden death, arteriosclerotic heart disease with congestive heart failure, and other.

For statistical analysis of age-adjusted data from the towns we used the official 1960 U.S. census data. The data that gave evidence of a remarkably low death rate from myocardial infarction among men in Roseto from 1955 to 1961 as compared to four neighboring communities and the United States at large, as shown in Figure 1.1, have been reported elsewhere, together with data on the surviving population as well[46] and are discussed in chapters 5 and 6. These findings have been widely cited as evidence for the positive effects of social cohesion and social support on longevity.[12, 47-52] Criticism concerning possible bias in the classification of the cause of death, and the procedures used to establish mortality rates, were published[53-55] and were rebutted.[56]

Expanded Study of Mortality

In order to compensate for the small numbers involved in the mortality data and for random fluctuations in the number of deaths in each town, the mortality data were expanded over a period of fifty years. All death records of inhabitants of Roseto and Bangor from 1935 to 1985 were obtained with the help of the Bureau of Vital Statistics in the Pennsylvania Department of Health and were examined and coded for cause of death. The results of this new study have been published[57] and are reported in chapter 5.

Clinical Study

A medical and sociological study of the inhabitants of Roseto, Bangor and Nazareth referred to in chapter 1 began with a preliminary two-week clinical survey of 10 percent of the population of Roseto in order to test the feasibility of conducting a larger study of the three towns. It was carried out in December 1962 by a team of twelve consisting of physicians, dieticians, and laboratory technicians.

The preliminary survey in Roseto was well attended, and the volunteer subjects were highly cooperative, enabling us to perform a full scale medical and sociological survey of Roseto the following summer. Bangor, immediately adjacent to Roseto, and Nazareth, a town eight miles distant from Roseto, were selected as controls. A 44-member team from the University of Oklahoma participated in the full-scale study, beginning in June 1963: an administrative director; ten physicians, including the director of the University of Oklahoma Biostatistical Center; three senior dieticians with six dietary students; one senior medical sociologist, assisted by a group of six graduate students in sociology; a clinical pathologist; a biochemist and two technicians; an electrocardiographic technician; and twelve medical students. Each community provided volunteer receptionists and coordinators.

Men and women over age 24 were recruited through announcements in the newspaper and through word-of-mouth promotion by helpful citizens in each community. In order to minimize possible bias in data obtained on a volunteer population, we gathered as controls a random sample of those over twenty-four years of age in Roseto and Nazareth who had not participated in the study. Thirty-six of 71 from the Roseto control list and 201 of 364 from the Nazareth list agreed to submit to examination. No significant differences between volunteer and random sample populations were found regarding the prevalence of evidence of the diseases studied, except that no persons with myocardial infarction were found in the random sample from Roseto or Nazareth. In view of the similarity of the samples, the data from the nonvolunteer group were included in the analyses.

The examinations were carried out in a local school building during the summers of 1963 to 1966. Roseto was studied first, then, during the summer of 1964, immediately adjacent Bangor, which, as already noted, shares its water supply with Roseto and is served by the same doctors and hospitals, and finally Nazareth in 1965. The participants, men and women over age 24, were examined with a careful history and physical examination including weight and height. Each person was questioned concerning dietary, smoking, and drinking behavior and participated in a structured sociological interview lasting about forty minutes. Also included were a 12-lead ECG; a blood sugar, hematocrit, serum cholesterol, triglycerides; and lipoprotein electrophoresis; clotting time; prothrombin time; fibrinolytic activity; and fibrinogen concentration. The examination areas were equipped with screened-in rooms, which, along with adjoining classrooms, were used for taking medical histories, dressing and examination, the sociological interview, getting the dietary, smoking, and drinking behavior histories, electrocardiograms, and laboratory tests on whole blood and serum samples. The receptionists and record keepers were supervised by the administrative director.

The patients provided the names and addresses of their grandparents, parents, children, and grandchildren, together with other identifying information including the cause and age of death, if known, of deceased family members. The latter were checked and the diagnoses verified by examining their actual death certificates (see chapter 5). The entire data gathering process during the survey consumed approximately two and a half hours.

The Samples

Table 4.1 lists by age and sex the populations and study samples from each town. Two hundred sixty-nine, or 57 percent of the 472 men, and 271, or 50 percent of the 544 women, in the population of Roseto over age 24 at the time of the 1962-63 survey participated in the full clinical (medical and sociological) examinations.

To enlarge and enhance the sociological data, the sociologists visited families in their homes (86 percent of the households) and interviewed the available members who had not already participated in the sociological interview.

In Bangor, 487 men and 640 women, 28 percent and 32 percent respectively, of the population over age 24 were included, as were 660 men and 789 women, 35 percent and 38 percent respectively, of the Nazarenes over age 24.

Non-Resident Relatives of Rosetans

In order to gauge social and health differences between Rosetans and their relatives who had not grown up in their ethnically homogeneous environment, we placed in one category those who had spent their entire lives in Roseto together with those who had been born and brought up in Roseto and had maintained their close ties there but were not resident at the time of the first survey because of schooling, employment, marriage, and so on. They were compared to their relatives living in Bangor or other nearby communities who had neither been born nor brought up in Roseto. Another comparative group consisted of relatives of Rosetans who lived

TABLE 4.1

Representatives of Clinic Samples in Roseto, Bangor, and Nazareth with Respect to Age and Sex

Age Group	ROSETO 1960 Population	ROSETO % of Population	ROSETO Total Clinic Sample	ROSETO % of Sample	BANGOR 1960 Population	BANGOR % of Population	BANGOR Total Clinic Sample	BANGOR % of Sample	NAZARETH 1960 Population	NAZARETH % of Population	NAZARETH Total Clinic Sample	NAZARETH % of Sample
Males												
25-34	109	23	63	23	293	17	88	18	400	22	123	19
35-44	121	26	60	22	380	22	96	20	406	22	142	21
45-54	102	22	63	23	430	25	139	29	410	22	161	24
55-64	69	15	43	16	307	18	85	17	307	17	130	20
65+	71	15	40	15	305	18	76	15	314	17	104	16
Totals	472		269	57	1,715		487	28	1,837		660	36
Females												
25-34	118	22	55	20	323	16	87	14	405	20	143	18
35-44	143	26	66	24	477	24	144	23	454	22	178	23
45-54	145	27	80	29	458	23	170	26	440	21	175	22
55-64	64	12	48	18	348	17	117	18	365	18	169	21
65+	75	14	22	12	405	20	122	19	386	19	124	16
Totals	544		271	57	2,001		640	32	2,050		789	38

Note: Only individuals age 25 and over were examined in the clinics.

in nearby states such as Connecticut, Maryland, Florida, Ohio, and New York who identified themselves sufficiently with Roseto to regularly attend the annual July festival of Our Lady of Mt. Carmel. We recruited as many of them as possible to participate in the medical and sociological survey. They were helpful for comparison because, although these relatives were emotionally tied to the community, their social environment differed sharply from that of Roseto.

The population of Bangor was divided into four wards. The Roseto family members who lived in Bangor identified themselves in varying degree with Roseto. The Fourth Ward, located on the edge of Roseto and immediately adjacent to the church of Our Lady of Mt. Carmel, is populated predominantly by Italian families that, like those in Roseto, trace their origin to Roseto Val Fortore, most of whom think of themselves as Rosetans. Fifty-one men and 80 women, making a total of 131 people from the Fourth Ward, participated in the first survey. Twenty-four men and 37 women, making a total of 61 people over the age of 24, participated in both surveys. Twenty people, all women, missed the second survey; 27 men and 23 women, making a total of 50 people, died in the interim between surveys.

Of the 290 men and 327 women who were examined in the 1962-63 survey, 40 percent of the men and 22 percent of the women had died before 1985. Of those still living in 1985, only 32 percent of the men and 35 percent of the women participated in the 1985 survey. The number of participants among Rosetans, Bangor's Fourth Ward inhabitants, and Roseto relatives living elsewhere is shown in table 4.2.

One hundred sixty Roseto men and 194 Roseto women not included in the 1962-63 survey were nevertheless visited in their homes and were administered the sociological interview in 1966, as were a few relatives serving in Bangor's Fourth Ward and elsewhere. Similarly, home interviews were conducted among 86 men and 129 women who failed to participate in the 1985 survey.

The 1985 Follow-Up Medical and Sociological Survey

In collaboration with the medical sociologists John Bruhn and Bill Philips and a group of physician's assistants from the School of Allied Health Sciences of the University of Texas Medical Branch in Galveston, a second thorough medical and sociological examination of individual

Rosetans was undertaken in the same school house and in essentially the same fashion as before. Limited financial support at this time precluded our repeating the physical examinations and testing in Bangor and Nazareth, but with the collaboration of the Center for Social Research at Lehigh University, Bethlehem, Pennsylvania, sociological interviews were carried out during visits to households in both Roseto and Bangor. Thus, not only were the Rosetans who participated in the first survey compared to themselves twenty-three years later but also to new groups of Rosetans in age decades that correspond to those in the original study. Although the 1985 clinical observations were restricted to Roseto, the 1985 home visits for sociological interviews were conducted in both Roseto and Bangor.

TABLE 4.2

	First Survey		Both Surveys		Died Between		Missed 2nd		2nd Survey Only	
	M	F	M	F	M	F	M	F	M	F
Rosetans	290	327	118	165	117	73	55	89	42	39
Fourth Ward	62	80	25	39	27	23	10	18	3	3
Relatives	205	182	60	53	67	40	78	89	97	110

Note: Includes the randomly selected controls plus a few whose addresses were corrected because they had originally supplied thier business or school rather than home address.

Social Structure and Characteristics of the Community

From 1964 to 1977 one of the authors (Stewart Wolf) visited Roseto and Bangor several times each year to observe and record social changes. In late 1977 he moved permanently to a locality within five miles of Roseto and Bangor. Thereafter, the two towns were under more or less continuous scrutiny. In view of this participation in the life of both communities, attending weddings, funerals, family dinners, backyard cook-outs, and special festivals, the author was virtually in the situation of a participant observer.

In 1962 Roseto celebrated its Golden Jubilee, the Fiftieth anniversary of the town's incorporation; the Seventy-Fifth anniversary, the Diamond Jubilee, took place in 1987. Both festivals were attended by participants in the study. The commemorative books published for each occasion provided useful data on the history of Roseto and reflected the local color and changing customs of the community.

A more systematic and quantifiable inquiry into social changes in the two communities was launched in 1985 by an independent group, the Center for Social Research at Lehigh University. Designed to document changes in local institutions, religious, commercial, social, and political changes-it addressed issues such as decisions in the selection of marital partners, church attendance, voting patterns, level of education, type of job held, immigration and emigration, purchase of new automobiles and homes and involvement in outside social, religious, and political activities (see chapter 7).

Long-Term Study of Major Roseto Clans

In 1962 there were 207 family names in Roseto. Many families had produced four new generations since the original immigration. A young woman who had acquired a new name through marriage might identify herself primarily with the family of her husband, or her husband might become a part of the family of her parents. In this fashion clans were formed and perpetuated.

From the sociological interviews it was possible to learn which families were generally considered to represent clans. The criteria included the large size of family; the family having immigrated to Roseto during the early years, preferably from Roseto Val Fortore or adjoining towns; their degree of participation in community affairs; and evidence that family members were willing to sacrifice to provide for relatives in need. Although the main concern of family clans was for parents, grandparents, and children-especially for the education of the children-their obligation extended beyond the nuclear family, even to distant relatives. With all available relatives and even neighbors, the clans celebrated all of life's landmarks: births, first communion, graduation at each level of schooling, engagement, marriages, birthdays, and anniversaries. Some of the clans held reunions every few years, to which they drew members from all over the United States, Canada and even Italy.

Hypothesis

Roseto's stable structure, with its emphasis on family cohesion and the mutually supportive attitudes of its people together with its remarkably low mortality rate from myocardial infarction from 1955-1961 and low prevalence of coronary heart disease during the early 1960s had led us to the hypothesis that salutary human relationships had contributed to the relative immunity of its inhabitants to myocardial infarction.

The procedure for testing the hypothesis was arranged in such a way as to deal first with the relatively uncontaminated issue of total mortality in the two towns, Roseto and Bangor, that share the same environment, water supply, doctors, and hospitals. The objectives, design, and results of that study are presented in chapter 5. In order to determine whether or not genetic influences or social forces from clan membership might be involved, we looked for clustering of fatal myocardial infarction or congestive heart failure due to coronary heart disease in certain families. The objectives, design and result of the mortality study are also to be found in Chapter 5.

Alternate Hypotheses

A. Biased Data

1. The data comparing Roseto and Bangor may be skewed by a different diagnostic style among physicians serving Roseto versus those serving Bangor.

Control. The two immediately adjacent towns have coextensive streets and were served by the same physicians and local hospitals.

2. The samples examined may not be representative of the population itself.

Control. Random samples solicited and examined during the early survey were found to be closely comparable to the voluntary participants in terms of health and social attitudes. The mortality data was, of course, not susceptible to selection bias since all death certificates were obtained and examined.

3. The differences observed could be attributable to different mineral content of the drinking water.

Control. Roseto and Bangor shared the same water supply.

4. The lower mortality from, and prevalence of, myocardial infarction in Roseto as compared to Bangor may be explained by the out-migration of the susceptible inhabitants.

Control. In the prospective study of the town age adjusted mortality from myocardial infarction actually increased despite any out-migration.

B.Genetic Factors

The reason for the low mortality from myocardial infarction in Roseto may have been that the immigrants from Italy came from an unusually hardy stock with little susceptibility to coronary heart disease. Thus the increased death rate from myocardial infarction in Roseto may have been primarily a result of the original gene pool of Rosetans being diluted by intermarriage with non-Rosetans and non-Italians.

Control. While the possible effects of dilution of the original gene pool could not be altogether eliminated, we attempted to challenge such an assumption by correlating year of birth (beginning in 1880 and extending to 1960) with the year of each subject's first myocardial infarction. Correlation was also made between each subject's age and the year of his or her first myocardial infarction, and between the year of birth and the subject's age at his or her first myocardial infarction.

Since there were few spouses from outside Roseto among individuals born prior to 1920, and since their marriages would have occurred in around 1940 and their children would have been 40 years old in 1980, gene pool dilution would have had relatively little influence on coronary disease during the course of our study.

An additional test of this alternate hypothesis of favorable genetic endowment was made by comparing the prevalence of death from myocardial infarction in each succeeding generation of Rosetans, beginning with those born prior to 1882 and extending it four to six generations up to 1985.

All Rosetan inhabitants of Bangor's Fourth Ward and all Roseto relatives living elsewhere who had participated in one or both surveys and who had died of myocardial infarction or congestive heart failure due to coronary heart disease were linked with all members of their families who had died from any cause between 1925 and 1985. The results of this inquiry are described in chapter 6. The same population sample was used to relate age at death from myocardial infarction and congestive heart failure to decade of death. Four decades of relatively traditional social influences (1925-1964) were compared to the two later decades (1965-1985) that were characterized by rapid social change. These data are presented in chapter 6.

C. Dietary Considerations

Dietary change was responsible for the increased prevalence of, and mortality from myocardial infarction.

Control. Dietary behavior of Rosetans was achieved by comparing the data on dietary habits in Roseto among the participants of the first survey (1962-63) with those in the second (1985). The data, gathered in the fashion described earlier covered changes in cooking habits including use of lard, butter, and olive oil and the consumption of eggs and milk. The changes in dietary behavior were correlated with changes in prevalence of, and mortality from, myocardial infarction.

D. Other Risk Factors

Other coronary risk factors may have intervened during the period of study.

Control. Individual data on cholesterol concentration and the presence of diabetes, hypertension, and obesity were gathered on all subjects in Roseto and Bangor who participated in the first survey and were compared to the outcome during the follow-up period. The data are presented and analyzed in chapter 7.

E. Population Shift

The data cannot be evaluated because of a major change in the character of the population during the twenty-five-year interval.

Control. Those who had moved into the community during the interval between 1963 and 1985 were not included in the analysis.

F. Change in the Relationship of Causes of Death

The rising mortality in Roseto was due to a relative decrease in mortality attributable to other conditions such as infectious diseases, trauma, and emphysema.

Control. Mortality data were collected by examining all death certificates of Rosetans and Bangorians from 1935 to 1985 as described in chapter 5. The frequency of ten categories of cause of death was calculated over the sixty-year interval.

G. Changing Age of the Population

The increase in mortality in Roseto was attributable to the fact that in 1985 the average age of the population was higher than in 1963.

Control. The data gathered were not only corrected for age but were standardized with the data from Bangor. Moreover, the mortality statistics of succeeding generations of Rosetans and Bangorians were separately analyzed with respect to age at death, beginning in 1925 or 1935 and extending to 1985.

5

Mortality in Roseto and Adjacent Bangor, 1935-1985

As mentioned in chapter 1, the study of the Italian-American community of Roseto was prompted by the discovery that the mortality rate among men from myocardial infarction was approximately 50 percent of that in four neighboring communities.

Total mortality among men and women in Roseto (Population 1,630) had been compared with that in immediately adjacent Bangor (Population 5,766), which shared with Roseto the same water supply, physicians, and hospital services; Nazareth (Population 6,209), about ten miles southwest, and Stroudsburg (Population 6,070) and East Stroudsburg (Population 7,674) both located about ten miles north of Roseto. The populations of each town, divided into age and sex, are shown in table 5.1.

Death certificates of all people dying in the five towns between 1955 and 1961, obtained through the courtesy of the Bureau of Vital Statistics of the Department of Health of the Commonwealth of Pennsylvania, were reviewed and verified whenever possible from physician's and hospital records. The resulting values indicated a much lower death rate from myocardial infarction in Roseto than in the other four towns (table 5.2). This low death rate was particularly striking among Rosetan males as shown graphically in figure 1.1 of chapter 1.

The death rates from arteriosclerotic heart disease (without evidence of myocardial infarction), hypertensive heart disease, and other cardio-

TABLE 5.1
Population Distribution by Age and Sex of the Five Communities Studied, 1960 CENSUS

TOWN	SEX	<5	5-14	15-24	25-34	35-44	45-54	55-64	65>	TOTAL
Roseto	M	83	151	74	109	121	102	69	71	780
	F	70	153	83	118	143	145	63	75	850
Bangor	M	243	494	296	293	380	430	307	305	2,748
	F	226	414	367	323	477	450	348	405	3,018
Nazareth	M	289	536	321	400	406	410	307	324	2,983
	F	276	512	388	405	454	440	365	386	3,226
Stroudsburg	M	243	488	261	305	370	374	309	395	2,745
	F	279	479	422	328	378	443	415	581	3,325
E. Stroudsburg	M	351	653	748	403	439	399	347	347	3,687
	F	366	632	774	423	495	428	408	461	3,987

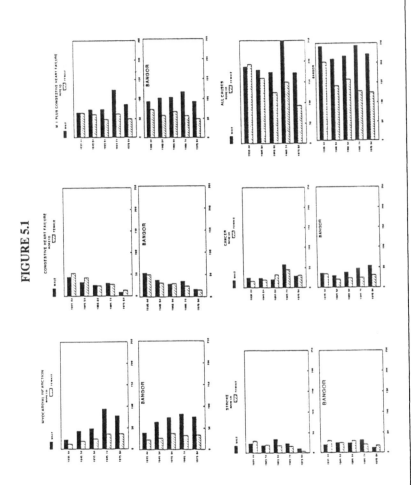

FIGURE 5.1

Death Rates/1000 in Roseto and Bangor from Various Causes Arranged According to Sex and Decade of Death

TABLE 5.2
Average Annual Death Rates per 100,000 from Myocardial Infarction by Age and Sex, 1955–1961

Town	Sex	Under 35	35–44	45-54	55-64	65-Up	Age * Adjusted
Roseto	M	—	—	144	—	813	109
	F	—	—	—	—	801	89
Nazareth	M	—	—	253	1,049	2,545	423
	F	—	—	134	234	1,309	186
Bangor	M	—	35	305	1,082	1,866	363
	F	—	58	64	368	1,431	212
Stroudsburg	M	42 (25–34)	74	373	910	1,980	378
E. Stroudsburg	M	—	32	284	705	2,344	374
	F	—	—	33	144	689	96

* Age adjustment performed by the direct method using the combined 1960 census male populations for the five communities as the standard population.

vascular causes were essentially similar for the five towns (table 5.3).[45] The death rate from all causes was extended from 1955 to 1963 and was found to be considerably lower in Roseto than in the other four towns, especially among males between the ages of 35 and 64, and males and females under age 55 (table 5.4).[46] At that time Roseto did not differ from its neighbors with respect to the usually accepted coronary risk factors, but except for Nazareth, it stood out from the others by virtue of close family ties and cohesive, mutually supportive behavior of its inhabitants.

TABLE 5.3
Average Annual Age-Adjusted Death Rates per 100,000 from Arteriosclerotic Heart Disease (Exclusive of Myocardial Infarction), Hypertension Heart Disease, and Other Cardiovascular Diseases by Sex 1955–1961

Town	Sex	Ashd (CHF)	HCVD	Other
Roseto	M	158	0	112
	F	89	22	44
Nazareth	M	161	31	97
	F	170	25	59
Bangor	M	137	5	114
	F	142	16	127
Stroudsburg	M	121	21	80
	F	66	29	37
E. Stroudsburg	M	128	24	79
	F	98	25	56

Nazareth had an even longer tradition of community cohesion in the United States. than did Roseto. As described in chapter 3, Nazareth, though no longer an exclusively Moravian community, was a town with high morale, close families, and a strong sense of identity. The association of these social characteristics with low coronary mortality suggested the hypothesis that social stability (secure, predictable social relationships) may be protective against heart attacks and conducive to longevity.

By the early 1960s there were indications of impending social change in Roseto.[21] Interviews with many of the towns people between 25 and

35 years of age and with the teenage group indicated that they were prepared to abandon, to a large extent, their old community ways in favor of the more typically American behavior of neighboring communities. We therefore predicted in 1963 that, should there be a loosening of its traditional values and behavior, Roseto's apparent relative protection from fatal myocardial infarction would be lost. A subsequent investigation of social change and mortality, extending the data from 1966 to 1970 and then to 1974 appeared to confirm this prediction,[27,21] although there remained a possible source of bias due to the small size of Roseto, discrepancies in the populations of the two towns, and the relatively short (twenty years) span of the study. An extension of the data was therefore undertaken in a new study conducted in collaboration with the Center for Social Research at Lehigh University involving Brenda Egolf, Judith Lasker, and Louise Potvin.

Reexamination and Extension of Data on Mortality in Roseto and Bangor

The mortality data on Roseto and Bangor were reaccumulated and extended to cover a span of fifty years, 1935-1984. All death certificates in Bangor and Roseto extending from 1935 to 1985 were obtained from the Bureau of Vital Statistics and individually studied. In order to obtain death certificates for those who may have died while out of town, we examined all obituary notices published between 1935 and 1985 in the local newspaper serving Roseto and Bangor, and in the newspaper in the county seat as well. The papers had listed not only virtually all the deaths in Roseto and Bangor identified for us by the death certificates, but also additional deaths of individuals who had died while visiting in nearby communities or out of state. The death certificates of those who had died in other localities in Pennsylvania, were obtained through the alphabetical listings of the Bureau of Vital Statistics of Pennsylvania and the certificates of those who had died out of state were obtained from the bureaus of vital statistics in New Jersey, Ohio, Connecticut, California, and Florida, where most of the deaths had occurred. A total of 3,859 certificates was thereby assembled.

Diagnostic Criteria

The criteria for the diagnosis of death from myocardial infarction included all instances where myocardial infarction was listed on line 1 of the certificate, "immediate cause of death" or when sudden death was listed on that line and myocardial infarction, ischemic heart disease, arteriosclerotic cardiovascular disease, coronary heart disease, or similar phrases appeared on the next "due to," lines of the death certificate.

The diagnosis of congestive heart failure was made when that diagnosis appeared on line 1 or two associated with chronic ischemic heart disease, chronic myocarditis, cardiomyopathy, and similar phrases appearing as "due to" or contributing cause.

Cancer was diagnosed when cancer, Ca, or carcinoma appeared on either the "immediate cause of death" line, the "due to" line, or "contributing causes" line.

Stroke was diagnosed when CVA, stroke, cerebral hemorrhage, or thrombosis appeared on the "immediate cause" line, with arteriosclerosis, atherosclerosis, or hypertension on one of the other lines.

Age Adjustment and Standardization

Tables 5.5 and 5.6 give the total population in various age groups in Roseto and Bangor, respectively, as listed by the U.S. Census Bureau from 1930 to 1980. Since the focus of our interest was coronary disease, age-adjusted rates were computed only for those aged thirty-five and older. Rates were based on ten-year averages over the period 1935-1985, using the five years on either side of an official census count, with the census figures as the denominator. A more fine tuned approach would have been to use five-year intervals, but reliable population estimates were not available between censuses for such small towns. Populations declined between 1930 and 1980 from 1,746 to 1,484 in Roseto, and from 5,824 to 5,006 in Bangor.[57] Moreover, in view of the relatively small number of annual deaths within any given age by sex category or for any particular cause of death, rates computed over a five-year period might be misleading.

Mortality rates in the two towns were standardized for age, using the sum in each age group in Roseto and Bangor in 1940 as the standard population. Total death rates were computed as well as separate rates from myocardial infarction, congestive heart failure, stroke, and cancer. The ratio of Roseto to Bangor rates was then calculated, and statistical significance was assigned to differences at the 95 percent confidence level.[57]

FIGURE 5.2

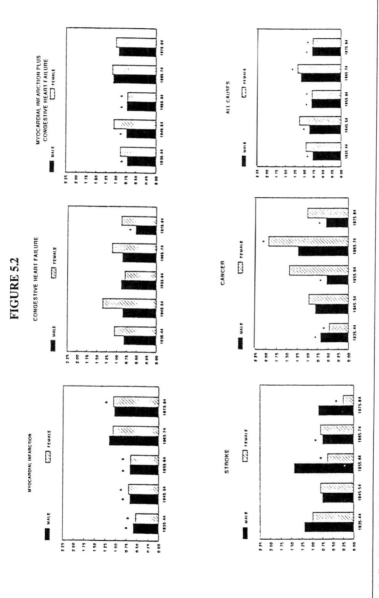

Standardized Mortality Ratios, Roseto/Bangor with Confidence Levels

* = 95 percent confidence

FIGURE 5.3

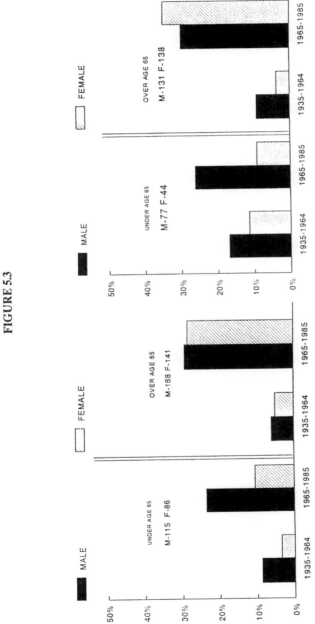

Deaths from Myocardial Infarction as a Percentage of All Deaths.

Note: The total male and female deaths (all causes) is shown in the center of each panel.

Results

Figure 5.1 provides age-adjusted specific and total mortality rates for the two communities over the course of five decades. Overall mortality for Bangor men remained fairly stable but declined over the sixty-year span among Bangor women and Roseto men and women. Deaths from cancer increased over the years in Roseto men and women, but no clear trend among Bangor men and women was described. Fatal stroke varied unevenly among all four groups.

The mortality rate for myocardial infarction among Roseto men and women was initially very low but showed a progressive rise over the entire thrity-year period (1935–1964). The rate for men in Bangor, which also rose, remained significantly higher than that in Roseto. In the decade 1965–1974 there was a sharp increase in coronary mortality among Roseto men and women. When deaths from congestive heart failure were added to those from myocardial infarction there was a significantly lower mortality rate among Roseto men than among Bangor men during the years prior to 1965. After 1965 the rate of coronary mortality rose sharply in Roseto approximating that in Bangor. The increase was less marked among women than men.[58]

Figure 5.2 shows the same data as figure 5.1, but expressed as the Roseto-to-Bangor ratio of mortality rates. The data on deaths from myocardial infarction, myocardial infarction plus congestive heart failure and total deaths are shown graphically in figures 5.2 to 5.4.

These findings, which cover a span of fifty years, have confirmed the earlier inference based on a shorter period of study that the Roseto death rate from myocardial infarction was significantly lower than that in immediately adjacent Bangor prior to 1965. The 1965 spurt of coronary deaths occurred at a time when the predicted decrease in social cohesion in Roseto became clearly manifest[27,58]. As described in detail in chapter 7, there had been a rapid and radical social change in Roseto. The earlier beliefs and behavior that characterized the community and that were expressed in the family-centered social life had changed. The former tradition that encouraged the avoidance of ostentation, even among the affluent, intraethnic marriages, and nearly exclusive patronage of local businesses had faded. The behavior of Rosetans had changed toward the more familiar pattern of neighboring communities. No longer were new families living in three-generation households with a strong commitment

TABLE 5.4
Average Annual Death Rates per 1,000 from All Causes by Age and Sex for Roseto, Bangor, Nazareth, Stroudsburg, and East Stroudsburg 1955–1963

AGE GROUP	ROSETO		BANGOR		NAZARETH		STROUDSBURG		E. STROUDSBURG	
	Pop.* Av.	Rate	Pop.* Av.	Rate	Pop.* Av.	Rate	Pop.* Av.	Rate	Pop.* Av.	Rate
Male										
<5	83	1.34	243	6.86	289	7.69	243	9.60	351	6.96
5–14	151	.74	494	.67	536	.41	488	.23	653	.68
15–24	74	1.50	296	1.88	321	1.38	261	2.13	748	.59
25–34	109	—	293	2.66	400	.56	305	2.19	403	1.93
35–44	121	1.83	380	3.51	406	3.01	370	5.10	439	2.53
45–54	102	3.26	430	6.46	410	7.32	374	11.29	399	10.30
55–64	69	14.49	307	24.61	307	21.36	309	26.97	347	25.62
>65	71	64.17	305	70.68	314	95.89	395	75.95	347	79.73
Age-Adjusted Rates		9.72		13.00		15.22		14.83		14.24
Female										
<5	70	1.58	226	4.92	276	3.22	279	7.17	366	6.98
5–14	153	—	414	.54	512	.43	479	.23	632	.88
15–24	83	1.34	367	.60	388	.57	422	.53	774	.57
25–34	118	—	323	.34	405	1.10	328	1.35	423	2.36
35–44	143	.78	477	2.33	454	2.94	378	3.23	495	2.69
45–54	145	3.83	458	3.88	440	6.82	443	5.27	428	3.89
55–64	63	10.58	348	11.81	365	12.18	415	12.32	408	12.25
>65	75	47.41	405	59.53	386	68.22	581	53.74	461	56.88

FIGURE 5.4

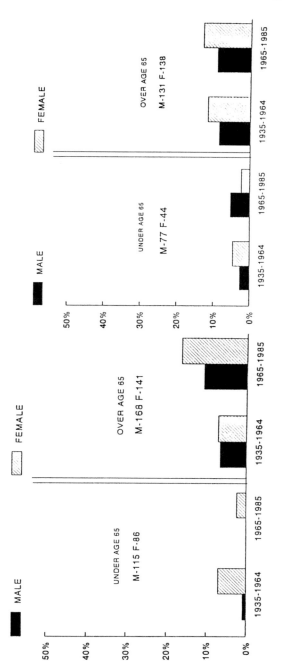

Deaths from Congestive Heart Failure (Arranged as in Figure 5.3)

to religion and to traditional values and practices. Family members appeared less cohesive and more materialistic, more "Americanized." Their attitudes were reflected in the statements made by Rosetans, old and young, during the sociological interviews, the results of which are discussed in the next chapter and in chapter 8.

Deaths from MI and CHF among Roseto Families

In order to detect evidence of clustering of coronary heart disease among certain Roseto families, which might suggest genetic or social influences on the distribution of coronary artery disease, all individuals who had participated in one or both of the surveys and had died of myocardial infarction between 1962 and 1985 were grouped with their family members who had died of any cause between 1925 and 1985. Cause of death, age at death, and year of death of parents, grandparents, siblings, children, and other blood relatives of the proband were recorded. A total of 283 men and 227 women from 118 families in Roseto constituted the group.

Clustering of fatal coronary heart disease in families was considered manifest if more than 50 percent of all deaths of family members were due to myocardial infarction or congestive heart failure. Such clustering of coronary deaths was identified among nine of eighty-five Roseto families. There were nine deaths from MI or CHF among fourteen total deaths in one family, seven among twelve in another, four among five deaths in three others, three among four in two others, and two among three in two others. Less than 50% of the total deaths in the remaining 109 families were due to either MI or CHF.

In view of the weak evidence of clustering of coronary mortality among these Roseto families, we examined the relationship of fatal myocardial infarction to time of death and age at death.

Figure 5.3 and 5.4 compare deaths from myocardial infarction and from congestive heart failure, respectively, among the Rosetan probands and their relatives with deaths among Bangor probands and their relatives. The rate of such deaths during the interval 1925-1964 are contrasted with the rate after 1965, arranged among individuals below and above 65 years of age. Eighteen percent of the Bangor probands were relatives of Roseto families. The increased number of deaths and their occurrence at a younger age after 1965 is clearly evident in both Roseto

TABLE 5.5
Roseto Population Census by Age and Sex

Age Group	1980 Male		1980 Female		1970 Male		1970 Female		1960 Male		1960 Female		1950 Male		1950 Female		1940 Male		1940 Female	
	N	%	N	%	N	%	N	%	N	%	N	%	N	%	N	%	N	%	N	%
<5	51	3.43	30	2.02	46	2.99	43	2.79	83	5.09	70	4.29	88	5.25	65	3.87	57	3.20	69	3.88
5-14	92	6.19	72	4.85	141	9.17	122	7.94	151	9.26	153	9.38	107	6.38	123	7.33	174	9.78	154	8.66
15-24	111	7.47	110	7.41	114	7.42	120	7.81	74	4.53	83	5.09	133	7.92	147	8.77	207	11.64	223	12.54
25-34	112	7.54	90	6.06	57	3.71	68	4.42	109	6.88	118	7.23	157	9.36	171	10.20	167	9.39	209	11.75
35-44	57	3.84	77	5.18	90	5.85	111	7.22	121	7.42	143	8.77	125	7.45	165	9.84	99	5.56	92	5.17
45-54	93	6.26	105	7.07	109	7.09	139	9.04	102	6.25	145	8.89	83	4.95	79	4.71	60	3.37	64	3.59
55-64	90	6.06	121	8.15	95	6.18	126	8.20	69	4.23	63	3.86	44	2.62	65	3.87	58	3.26	60	3.37
65>	105	7.07	168	11.30	67	4.36	88	5.27	71	4.35	75	4.60	67	3.99	57	3.40	45	2.53	40	2.24
	711	47.09	733	52.10	719	46.80	817	53.20	780	47.90	850	52.10	804	48.00	872	52.00	867	48.70	911	52.20
Total # Both Sexes	1,484				1,536				1,630				1,676				1,778			

TABLE 5.6
Bangor Population Census by Age and Sex

Age Group	1980 Male N	%	1980 Female N	%	1970 Male N	%	1970 Female N	%	1960 Male N	%	1960 Female N	%	1950 Male N	%	1950 Female N	%	1940 Male N	%	1940 Female N	%
<5	158	3.15	142	2.83	170	3.13	178	3.28	243	4.21	226	3.91	245	4.04	249	4.11	185	3.25	161	2.83
5-14	349	6.97	290	5.79	433	7.98	397	7.31	494	8.56	414	7.18	414	6.84	404	6.67	394	6.92	389	6.84
15-24	364	7.27	381	7.61	392	7.22	359	6.61	296	5.13	367	6.36	373	6.16	379	6.26	517	9.09	566	9.95
25-34	380	7.59	362	7.23	261	4.81	280	5.16	293	5.08	323	5.60	451	7.45	527	8.71	478	8.40	512	9.00
35-44	208	4.15	240	4.79	252	4.64	285	5.25	380	6.59	477	8.27	478	7.90	520	8.59	383	6.78	394	6.93
45-54	215	4.29	281	5.61	351	6.47	438	8.07	430	7.45	458	7.94	383	6.33	386	6.38	345	6.06	374	6.57
55-64	298	5.95	384	7.67	367	6.58	443	8.16	307	5.32	348	6.03	291	4.80	349	5.76	263	4.62	272	4.78
65>	347	6.93	607	12.12	330	6.08	499	9.19	305	5.28	405	7.02	273	4.51	328	5.42	225	3.95	229	4.02
Total # by Sex	2319	46.3	2687	53.7	2546	46.9	2879	53.1	2748	47.7	3018	52.3	2908	48.1	3142	51.9	2790	49.1	2897	50.9
Total # Both Sexes	5,006				5,425				5,766				6,050				5,687			

and Bangor and, by the chi-square method, is statistically significant for Roseto; P (P<0.01) for those under age 65 as well as for those over 65. The differences in Bangor are significant at that level only for those over age 65. The differences observed among deaths from congestive heart failure were less consistent and were not statistically significant.

A vivid example of the trend toward fatal myocardial infarction among the young in Roseto after 1965 occurred in the case of Mr. A., whose chest pains were first noted in 1961 and who died in 1971 at age 39. He was the first Rosetan to die of myocardial infarction under age 45. During the sociological interview conducted during the 1963 medical survey his personality and behavior were noted to deviate sharply from the traditional Rosetan pattern. He was restless, even reckless, generous but also self-indulgent and a heavy smoker.

He was born in Roseto, the oldest of four children, three brothers and one sister. In addition there were three half-brothers and five half-sisters from his mother's previous marriage. His father, a carpenter, had emigrated from Italy and had died at age 72 of aplastic anemia. His mother had diabetes and hypertension and died at 64 of myocardial infarction.

After graduating from high school he worked as a carpenter, and at 25 married a German girl 22 years old, also a high school graduate. He was Roman Catholic, and she converted to Catholicism. He described himself as a tense, nervous person who found it difficult to relax because, he said, "I feel I need to get things done and can't waste time."

Two years after the marriage he started his own construction business in a town about twenty miles away. He worked overtime and smoked three packs of cigarettes a day for twenty years. Neither he nor his wife was a member of any social or civic organization in Roseto. The marriage yielded four children. His wife resented the amount of time his work kept him from home. Her interest was in family life, his was in making money. His mother died when he was 28. It was for him "the most unhappy time in my life. I tried to lose myself in work." He said he had thought about moving away from Roseto "to get closer to my business."

He was first hospitalized for chest pains at age 29 when the construction business failed. After bankruptcy he founded a new company. This time the business succeeded financially, and, as he put it, he "lived like a king." He traveled to Puerto Rico, Las Vegas, gambled at the races, and bought expensive cars. He spent about a thousand dollars a week, gave wristwatches to his relatives' children, and responded generously to those who asked him for money or gifts without concern for repayment. He kept the problems of running the company to himself. His friend said: "You would never dream he had pressure on him unless you knew him. He always had it tough, but managed to get out of it." He enjoyed risk taking. Two months before his fatal heart attack, during a trip to Puerto Rico, he lost $9,000 in one night of gambling.

He was admitted to the intensive care unit of a local hospital for chest pains that started following his discovery that a bonding company had issued a fake bond in connection with a large contract. Upon being told his EKG was normal, he signed himself out of the hospital against medical advice and engaged in a poker game until the early hours of the morning. During the two weeks following his hospitalization, he made ten business trips to adjoining towns in addition to resolving the bonding problem. The day of his death he got into a fistfight with a drunk, was arrested, and was required to post a $1,000 cash bail bond. Later that day he attended the wake of a friend in a nearby city and, upon returning home, collapsed and died. He was 39 years old.

We are indebted to the American Public Health Association for permission to reproduce in this chapter material from the article "The Roseto Effect: A 50-Year Comparison of Mortality Rtes" by B. Egolf, J. Lasker, S. Wolf, and L. Potvin to be published in the August 1992 issue (vol. 82, no. 8) of the *American Journal of Public Health*.

ROSETO EVOLVING:
A Century in America

THE EARLY DAYS

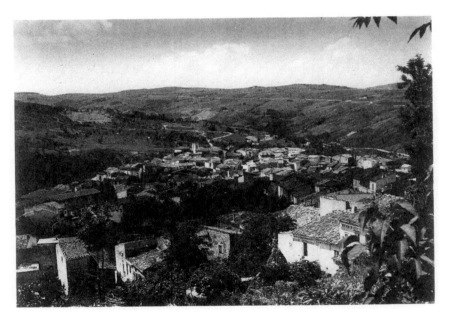

Former home, Roseto Val Fortore

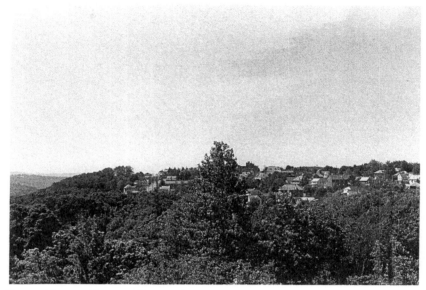

Present home, Roseto, Pennsylvania

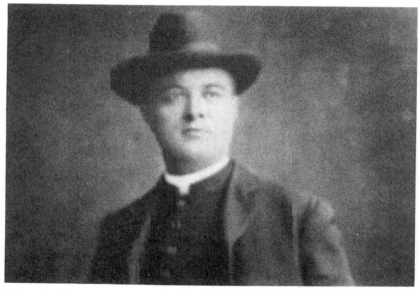

Father DeNisco came to serve a flock of bewildered and disorderly Italian immigrants. His influence built a cohesive and productive community

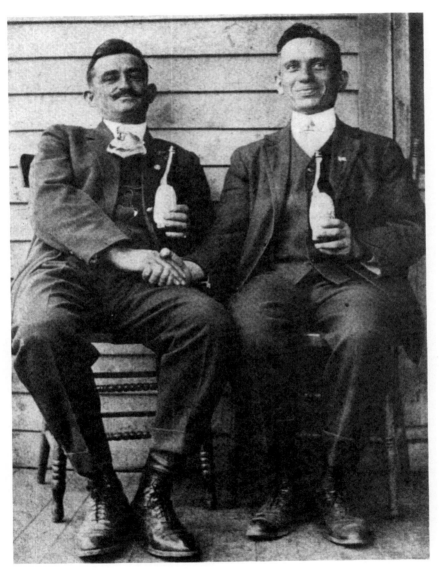

A restful moment for good friends

THEIR EARLY MEANS OF LIVELIHOOD

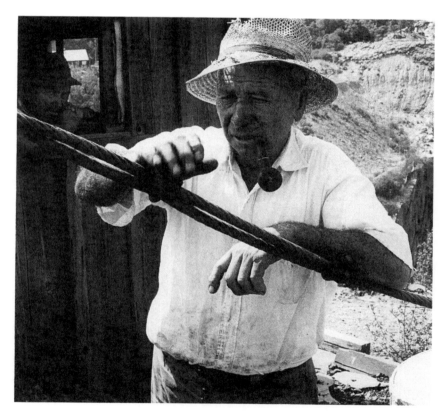

Directing the machinery that delivers the workers to the 200-foot-deep slate quarry pit

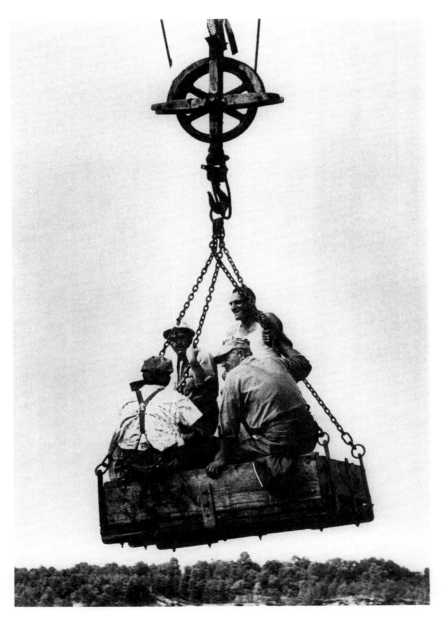

On the way down

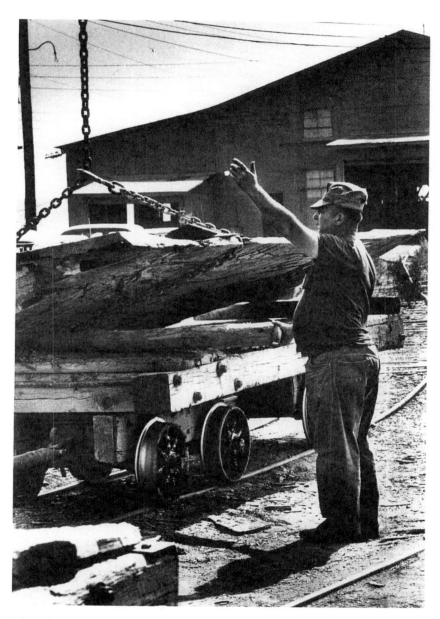

Directing a slab that will become roofing shingles

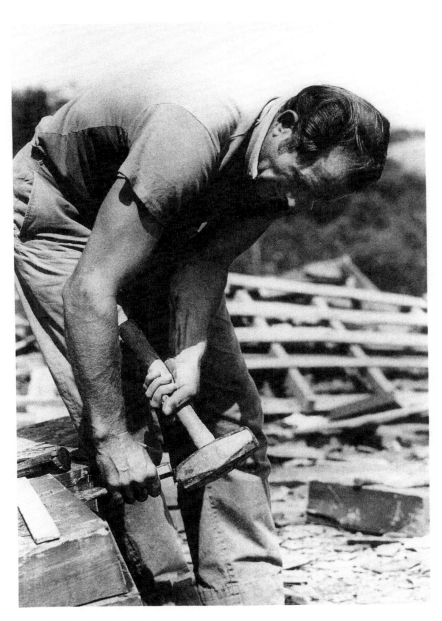

Skillfully splitting the slate

THE ANNUAL FESTIVAL OF OUR LADY OF MT. CARMEL

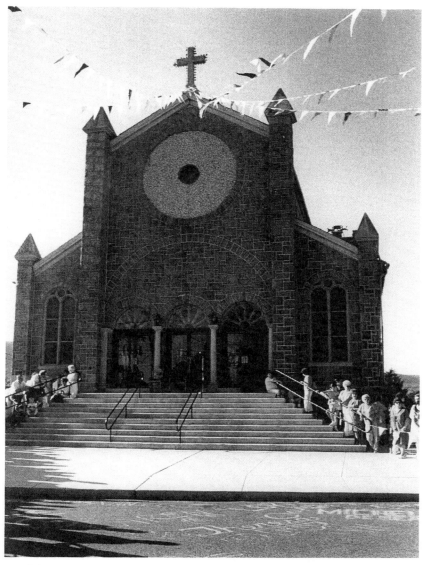

Awaiting the start of the procession at the church of Our Lady of Mt. Carmel

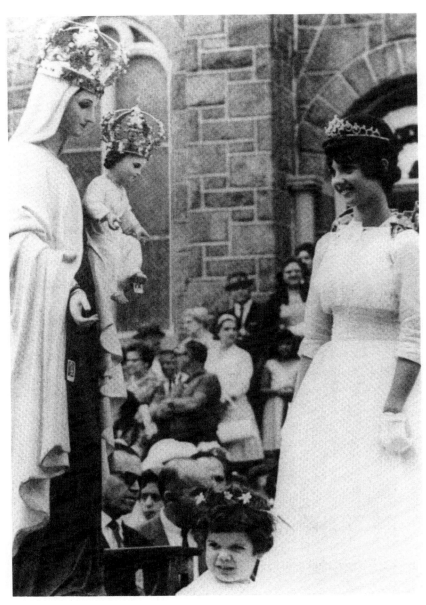

Amelia LeDonne with the Blessed Mother and Child

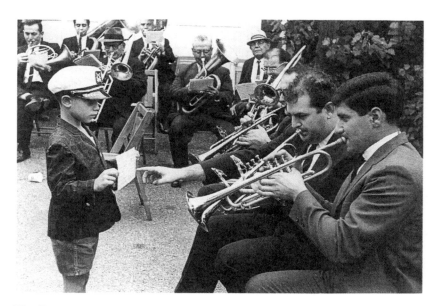

The Roseto Cornet Band tuning up

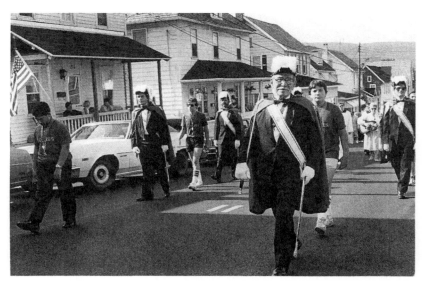

The Knights of Columbus

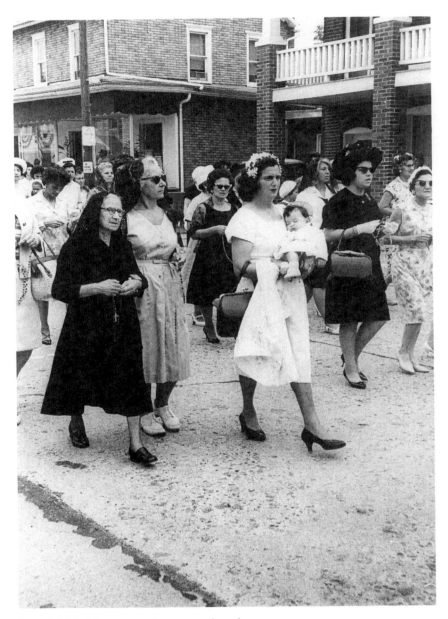

The faithful in procession repeating the rosary

WORKING ROSETANS

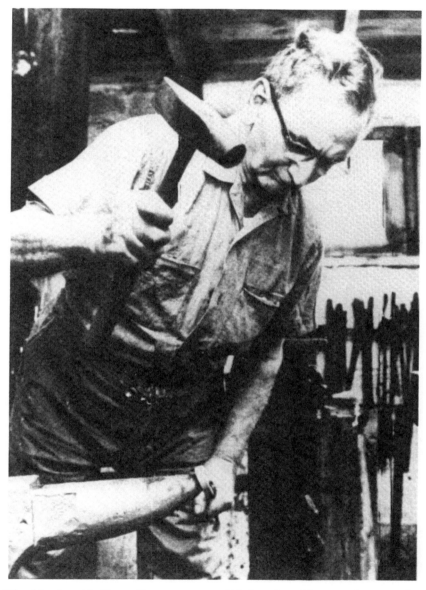

The blacksmith Peter Ronca, at age 86; he shoed horses from racing stables all over the eastern United States until his death at 94

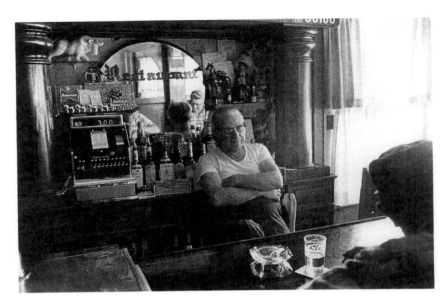

Mike Pacifico in his family's bar and restaurant that obtained the first liquor serving license in Roseto

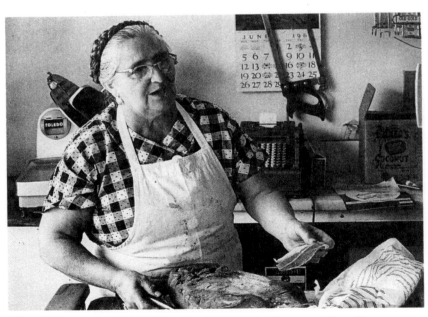

Teodoro DeFranco charming the customers at the butcher shop

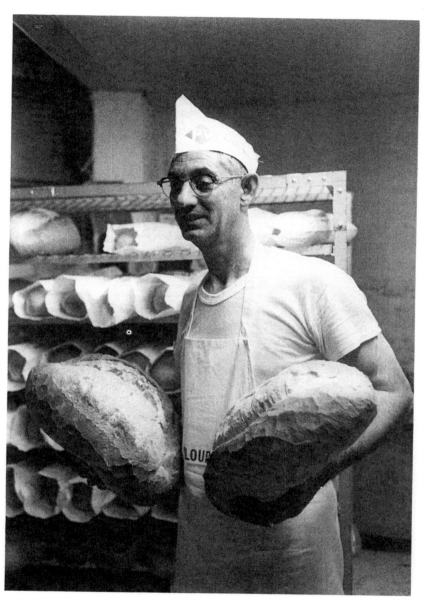

Matt LeDonne, the baker

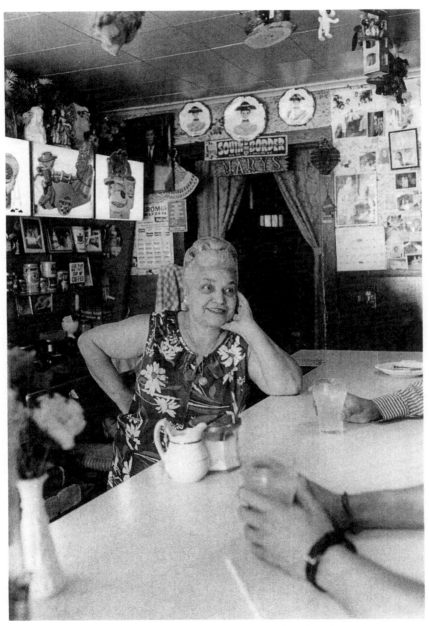

Mary Bert Cannavo encouraging the young at her luncheonette

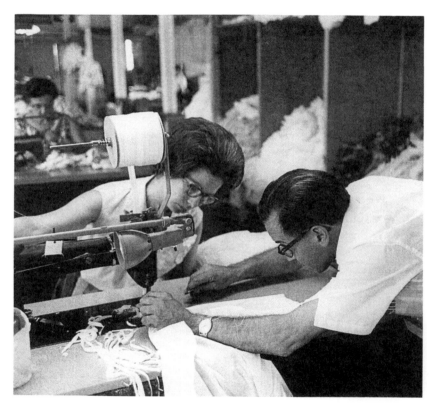

Textile finishing, a souce of income as the slate industry declined. Mayor
Giaquinto assisting one of his workers

THE LIFE OF THE TOWN

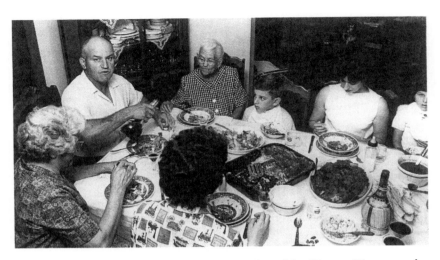

Four generations of the DeRea family at the table. Young Henry paying rapt attention to his grandfather Joe

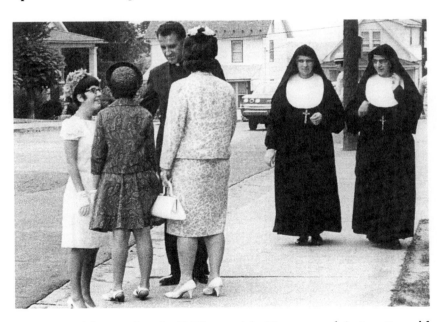

Father Renaldo greeting the DiPierro girls, Frances and Antonette, with their mother, Theresa. The nuns are Sister Superior Catherine and Sister Theresa

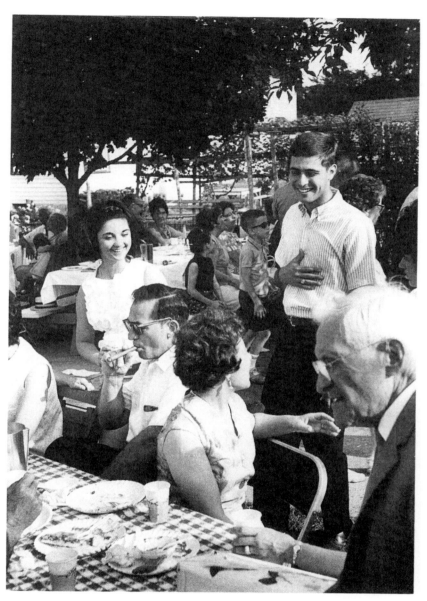

A multifamily backyard celebration

SOCIAL CHANGE

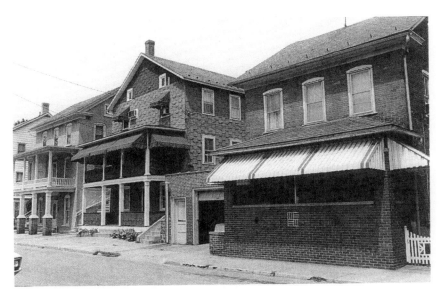

Garibaldi Avenue - 1963

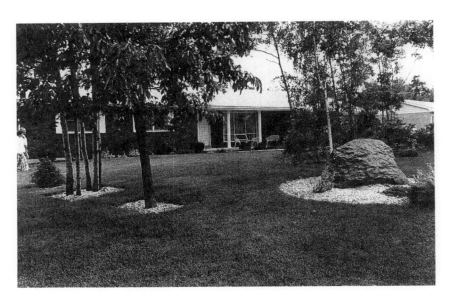

Kennedy Drive - 1975

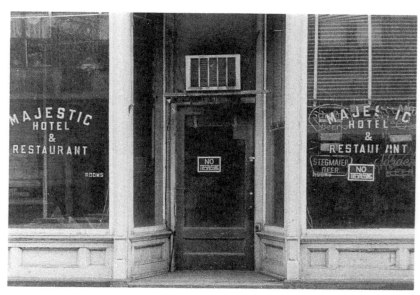

The former Majestic Hotel - 1980

CONTRASTING PERCEPTIONS FROM FOUR GENERATIONS OF THE ZITTO-CILIBERTI CLAN

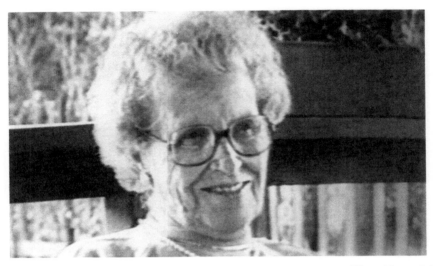

"Too much freedom—the girls and the boys—I no like, I'm old fashioned."

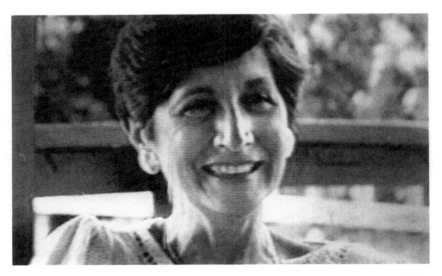

"Aren't all mothers that have their sons becoming doctors proud? I'm very proud of him."

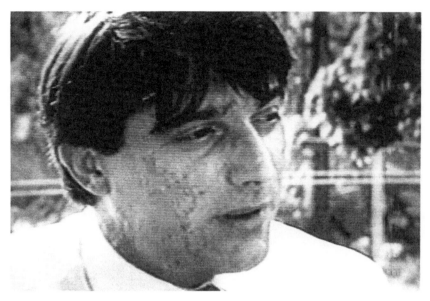

"We are very aggressive to get another job or to earn more money to attain a two-car family."

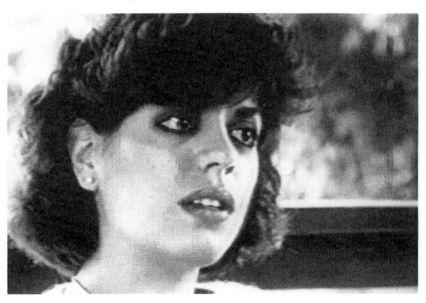

"I envy other people. I work hard so what I do have I'm proud of and I hope to be able to have more things. I worry about it—I'll be honest."

6

Changing Prevalence
of Myocardial Infarction 1962-1985

The previous chapter documented a sharp increase in Roseto's mortality rate from myocardial infarction that began about 1965. Not surprisingly, it was associated with a rise in manifestations of coronary artery disease among the living. The individual data from Roseto, Bangor, and Nazareth were reexamined in reference to the following criteria.

Diagnostic Criteria

The diagnosis of *myocardial infarction* was based on a history of one or more myocardial infarctions with survival documented in a hospital or by a physician or, in a few cases, by unequivocal evidence in the electrocardiogram of a "silent" myocardial infarction. Angina pectoris was identified by a typical history of pain (confirmed by a physician) with or without treatment by coronary artery bypass. The criterion for diagnosing *congestive heart failure* attributable to ischemic heart disease depended on a symptomatic history together with a physician's diagnosis and treatment with digitalis and/or diuretics.

The diagnosis of *hypertensive cardiovascular disease* was based on a history of treated hypertension and/or a resting diastolic blood pressure 95 mmHg at the time of examination.

The diagnosis of *diabetes* was made according to one or more of the following criteria:

1. History of diabetes treated with insulin, oral hypoglycemic agents, or diet.

2. A fasting blood sugar of 130 mg% or greater in the absence of a history of diabetes.

3. One-hour postprandial blood sugar of 180 mg% or greater.

4. Two-hour postprandial blood sugar of 150 mg% or greater.

5. Three-hour postprandial blood sugar of 130 mg% or greater.

6. Any blood sugar of 200 mg% or greater.

The diagnosis of *obesity* was made if body weight exceeded 120 percent of the "ideal" weight for the given age, height, and sex.

Subjects of Study

Table 4.2 in chapter 4 lists the numbers of Rosetans and their relatives in Bangor's Fourth Ward and elsewhere who participated in both the 1962-63 and the 1985 survey's as well as those who died between surveys, those who were alive but failed to attend the second survey, and those who participated in the second survey only. Four hundred sixty, or 40 percent of the 1,146 people examined in the first survey were available for follow-up more than twenty years later and were supplemented by 294 people who were studied in the second survey only.

Data from the Initial Survey

Among the 540 participants in the 1962-63 survey in Roseto, 16 men and 2 women had experienced a well-documented myocardial infarction. Two of the men, both under age 45, were still alive and well in 1991. Tables 6.1 and 6.2 display the number of infarcts encountered in Roseto and Bangor, the prevalence per 1,000, the number still surviving in 1990, and the causes of death of those who succumbed before 1991. Table 6.3 lists the percentage of those who had suffered myocardial infarction in Roseto and Bangor who also had other associated disorders. Figures 6.1-6.3 illustrate the timing of each subject's first myocardial infarction with reference to generation and age.

The serum cholesterol measurements made in 1962-63 on those who had experienced myocardial infarction were compared to the values

TABLE 6.1
Roseto 1962–63 Survey

Age at Survey	No. of Participants		M.I.		Prevalence		Alive in 1990		No. Dead		Cause of Death									
											M.I.		CHF		CVA		CA		Other	
	M	F	M	F	M	F	M	F	M	F	M	F	M	F	M	F	M	F	M	F
25–34	63	55																		
35–44	60	56																		
45–54	63	80	2		7.4		2													
55–64	43	48	9	2	33.5	7.4	1		8	2	5	1	1	1					2	
65+	40	32	5	0	18.6		1		4	2	4		1							
Total	269	271	16	2	59.5	7.4	4		12	2	9	1	1	1					2	

TABLE 6.2
Bangor 1962–63 Survey

Age at Survey	No. of Participants M	F	M.I. M	F	Prevalence M	F	Alive in 1990 M	F	No. Dead M	F	Cause of Death — M.I. M	F	CHF M	F	CVA M	F	CA M	F	Other M	F
25-34	54	60																		
35-44	59	101	3		9.2		2				1								1	
45-54	97	111	12	5	36.8	10.7	5	1	7	4	3	3					3	1	1	
55-64	57	98	10	2	30.7	4.3	5	1	5	1	2	1					1		1	
65+	59	96	15	15	46.0	32.2	5	4	10	11	4	2	2	2	2	5	2			2
Total	326	466	40	22	122.7	47.2	17	6	22	16	10	6	2	2	2	5	6	1	3	2

TABLE 6.3
Percentage of Those with Myocardial Infarctions Who Had Associated Disorders 1962–1965

	Hypertension	CHF	Diabetes	Obesity
Roseto	11.1	33.3	16.7	61.1
Bangor	25.8	24.2	4.8	40.3

obtained from a randomly selected age- and sex-matched group of Roseto participants. The mean serum cholesterol was 211 mg/dl among the patients and 220 among the controls. The highest cholesterol level for patients was 283 mg/dl and for controls, 252 mg/dl. Seven of the patients had higher concentrations of serum cholesterol than did controls. The cholesterol concentrations of the other eight were lower than their age- and sex-matched controls.

FIGURE 6.1
Roseto Myocardial Infarctions
1962–63 Survey

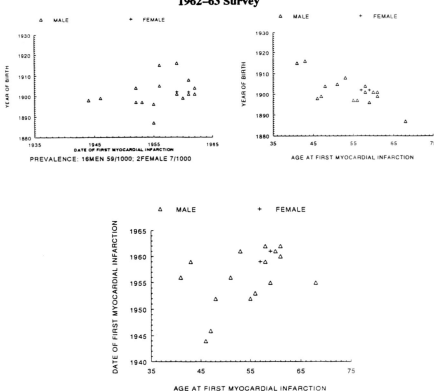

Reassessment in 1985

The 1985 follow-up examination was carried out in almost identical fashion to the initial study but, as explained in chapter 4, it focused only on Rosetans, their relatives living in Bangor's Fourth Ward (which, from an ethnic, geographic, and social perspective is virtually part of Roseto), and Roseto relatives from other sections of Bangor or elsewhere. Several subjects who had missed the first survey or were too young to have participated in it were examined in 1985, together with many of those who had attended the initial 1962-63 survey. Individuals who moved to Roseto between surveys and who were not members of Roseto families were not included in the analysis.

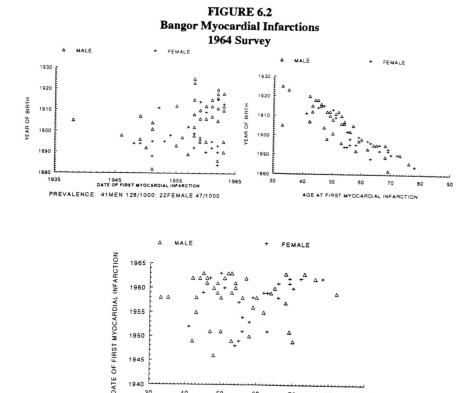

FIGURE 6.2
Bangor Myocardial Infarctions
1964 Survey

Table 6.4 displays, for the 1985 survey, the same data contained in tables 6.1 and 6.2.

Figure 6.4 compares the experiences of myocardial infarction among participants in Roseto during the 1985 survey with that of the inhabitants of the Fourth Ward and the other three wards of Bangor and elsewhere. It is evident that in all three communities, members of the younger generations were experiencing more myocardial infarctions than were documented in the original survey, and at an earlier age than their elders.

Associated Findings from the Sociological Interviews

The weakening of family cohesion and commitment to the community that became evident in about 1965 is documented in detail in the next chapter. It was apparent in the reduced attendance at our 1985 follow-up survey clinic. Although some families were intensely supportive, participated eagerly, and even helped with arrangements, some of those who had participated in the original study appeared indifferent and were unwilling to participate in 1985. During the 1962-63 survey, the clinic itself had been a vehicle for social intercourse. There was much less banter, gossiping, and friendly visiting during the subsequent survey in 1985.

The structured sociological interview administered in Roseto in both 1962-63 and 1985 included several questions of fact concerning family arrangements, interests, and activities of the respondents. Other questions sought opinions and judgments concerning the community, its qualities, leadership, family structure, children, the importance of religion, and so forth.

Replies to the early survey revealed a strong emphasis on the importance of the family and a close identification with the town and the community. Nevertheless, there were already indications of imminent change in the community from the replies on the questions in the sociological interviews conducted in the early 1960s. The inhabitants under age 35 seemed less committed than their elders to the traditional values and attitudes of Roseto. They expressed respect for them but manifested little interest in adopting what they considered to be "old fashioned ways." From group discussions with teenagers, the message was clear that they wanted to break away from the narrow, restricted environment of Roseto and join the American mainstream.

Although in 1962-63 the replies of parents indicated that the teenagers and young adult children were generally well behaved, they added such comments as: "Instead of working, they attend school longer.:" "The married ones have fewer children." "Children have too much leisure, can do anything they want, and have cars."

The 1985 parents, some of whom were teenagers at the time of the original study, complained that their children have too much freedom,

TABLE 6.4
Roseto 1985 Survey

Age at Survey	No. of Participants		M.I.		Prevalence		Alive in 1990		No. Dead		Cause of Death									
											M.I.		CHF		CVA		CA		Other	
	M	F	M	F	M	F	M	F	M	F	M	F	M	F	M	F	M	F	M	F
25-34	24	18																			
35-44	12	18	1		4.9		1														
45-54	34	46	3	1	14.6	3.8	3	1													
55-64	51	63	2	3	9.8	11.4	1	2	1	1		1			1						
65+	84	119	11	11	53.7	41.7	9	7	2	4		1	1	2					1	1	
Total	205	264	17	15	82.9	56.8	14	10	3	5		2	1	2	1				1	1	

are "spoiled," have too many material things, and lack respect for, and responsibility to, their elders. They expressed special concern about raising their own children in the currently permissive environment of the larger community surrounding Roseto.

FIGURE 6.3
Nazareth Myocardial Infarctions
1965 Survey

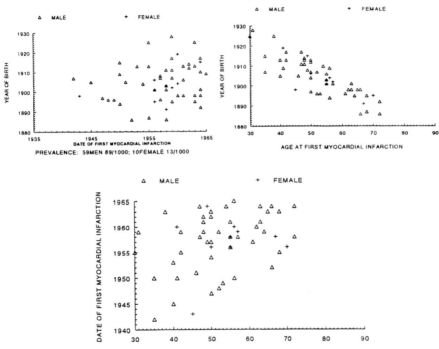

Their replies were similar to those of the older generations: "Today's children are less disciplined, lack respect, and have different morals." "Children today are lazy, have no religion or respect and too much freedom." "In Roseto there used to be a closeness, a respect for the elderly. You don't see much of that today." "There is more pressure on kids today. They try to keep up with the Joneses but the kids are not happy." "They get married and expect too much. The younger generation looks down on us for our lack of education."

FIGURE 6.4
Myocardial Infarctions
1985 Survey

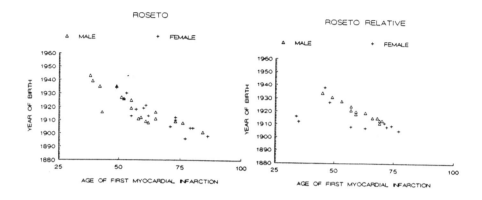

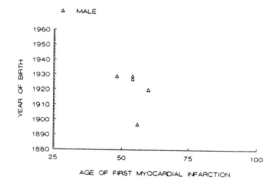

Paradoxically, informal discussions with Rosetans under age 25 during the summer of 1985 revealed an almost plaintive concern over the changing mores, the weakening of traditions, and the lack of equanimity among the inhabitants of Roseto.

The attitudes and perceptions of the participants in the 1985 survey grouped themselves to some extent according to age in roughly twenty-year cohorts.

Those Over 85 in 1985

All of those who were over 85 in the 1962-63 study, nearly all of whom had been born in Italy, had died. Those who were 63 or more at the time of the original survey and over 85 by 1985 included many people who had come to Roseto as young children with their parents, a few who had come over as youngsters without parents, and a few who had been born in Roseto before the turn of the century. Most of them spoke enthusiastically of the improvements in Roseto that had occurred long prior to our first visit; the development of roads, schools, churches, and clean neighborhoods with trees, gardens, and vineyards. As these changes were accompanied by more comfortable living circumstances and increasing prosperity, they also engendered new respect and social acceptance for the Italians. During their hard working years they had continued the tradition of the three generation household and had made sacrifices to educate their children but usually not beyond high school. These elderly people, now out of the mainstream of the community life were somewhat sheltered from the social changes and thus were able to maintain pretty well Roseto's traditional values and perspectives. Nevertheless, they expressed concern over the nonconforming social behavior of young adults, especially their extravagances, their relationships outside Roseto, and their lack of respect for their elders.

Those 46–65 in 1962–63 and 66–85 in 1985

Those in this age group had been the active shapers of the community during the original study twenty to twenty-five years earlier. Most of them referred with concern to the loosening of family ties and community cohesiveness during the interval since the original study. They were solicitous of, and attentive to, their parents, but instead of sharing the same house with them, most lived nearby or even next door. They had worked hard to provide college and often professional education for their children, but expressed ambivalence about the results, especially marriages to non-Italians and emigration to larger communities, some of them many miles away. Although proud of their children's achievements, the parents felt somehow victimized by them. Some even expressed a sense of guilt for having contributed to the changes in community values and attitudes. Nearly all acknowledged that Rosetans had become more mercenary and materialistic and less interested in religion and tradition. Although this cohort had experienced a low prevalence of clinical evidence of coronary artery disease (less than 0.005 of those examined), they were aware of and concerned about, the high prevalence (0.07) among the next generation (the cohort 46-65 in 1985), with their increased evidence of coronary artery disease in the form of angina pectoris and/or EKG abnormalities several had undergone coronary bypass surgery, or had even experienced a documented myocardial infarction.

Those 26–45 in 1962–63 and 46–85 in 1985

This generation was far removed from the struggles and self denial of the early days of Roseto and the painful social exclusion. Now, as the current leaders of the community, they were committed to "Americanization" with greater emphasis on competition than interdependence. Thus, they shared in shifting Roseto's focus from family to individual. Many of them had married non-Italians and had given their children nontraditional names. The ancient tabu against ostentation was nearly forgotten as they displayed their freedom to consume and enjoy the fruits of their wealth by shopping, traveling, and involving themselves in social activities outside of Roseto.

Those 6–25 in 1962-63 and 26–45 in 1985

As this generation, too young to have participated in the first survey, profited from the sacrifices of their parents and grandparents, many finished college and some had become physicians, dentists, or lawyers. Although they had spent a good deal of time with their grandparents in their early years during the period of rapid social change, most of them were frankly desirous of personal recognition, social power, and possessions, but they also expressed a longing for the old times: "The town is losing control, is losing pride." "Families are less close knit, spend less time together." "Neighbors no longer get together and drink coffee or talk." "Roseto has become more like Bangor—faster pace, people out for themselves." "People used to remain debt-free; now they worry about collection agencies." "There are no more small businesses—no more taverns or restaurants for people to relax." "People used to walk along the streets every evening and visit with one another, no more, too many cars." "Lower class, less disciplined people and dirty people are moving in." "Little Italy has become a league of nations."

Discussion

The analysis of mortality in Roseto reported in the previous chapter revealed a sharp rise in deaths from myocardial infarction beginning about 1965 and coinciding with a conspicuous social change from family-centered attitudes toward more self- centered, materialistic concerns among Rosetans. It is intriguing to try to relate the striking shifts in the social environment of Roseto to the equally impressive change in the death rate from coronary disease and in the prevalence of coronary disease among the living. The timing of the two events fits quite well our original hypothesis that social cohesion and cooperative attitudes were protective against coronary disease in Roseto and that contrary attitudes are destructive. If there is a causal relationship between their social values and practices and a low prevalence of coronary disease, the principal factor may reside in the uplifting and motivating effect on the human spirit afforded by close family ties, strong group attachments, strong sense of place, and a deep identification with the church. Chapter 8 will explore the possible impact of the loosening of such ties and the abandonment of traditions compared to the influence of other, more commonly cited factors predisposing to coronary heart disease.

Other Studies

Other investigators have offered evidence of the salutary effect of emotional support in an especially strong family and community structure. C. B. Thomas, in a long-term prospective study of Johns Hopkins medical students, found that the family values and relationships to which the students had been exposed as children could significantly predict subsequent coronary heart disease and other illnesses.[59-61]

Kaplan, Cassel, and Gore have marshaled evidence concerning the interaction between stressful circumstances and social support in the pathogenesis and prevention of several diseases.[62] They recommended as preventive strategies deliberate efforts in child rearing to encourage affiliations and interdependence, emphasis on building morale with relationships among workers in industrial settings, and recognition of the potential value of strong religious commitments.

In a study of blue-collar men who had lost their jobs in company shutdowns, Gore found that a low degree of family support further exacerbated the stress of unemployment. Men who were unemployed and unsupported showed significant increases and variations in serum cholesterol, illness symptoms, and depression over unemployed men who enjoyed a high degree of family support.[63]

James Lynch, who has examined the question of human companionship in relation to health and longevity, found that men and women living alone, especially if widowed or divorced, were at a significantly higher risk of early death.[12] In his intriguing book he offers a persuasive argument for the healthful quality of human dialogue and love.

Fuchs has called attention to the fact that two neighboring states, Nevada and Utah, are at opposite ends of the spectrum of mortality from myocardial infarction.[64] The ethnic mix of the two states is very similar, both are among the nation's highest in level of education and the urban-rural mix is about the same in the two states. The average per capita income in Nevada is 15 to 20 percent higher than in Utah. For men and women between the ages of 25 and 64, however, Nevada in 1960 had by far the highest death rate in the country. Utah had one of the lowest. Although the Mormon ban on drinking and smoking may be an important factor, Fuchs speculates that the stability of social structure and the close family ties in Utah may play an important role in the discrepancy between the two states with respect to mortality from ischemic heart disease. Nevada's social structure is marked by fractured and disrupted family relationships.

A similar hypothesis to explain why Japan has enjoyed one of the lowest rates of coronary heart disease in the world was set forth by Matsumoto.[65] Not only are family relationships extremely close and mutually supportive, but the job situation is in sharp contrast to that in our country. Matsumoto describes the nature of the employer-employee relationship in Japan as bilateral commitment. Being hired by a Japanese firm is like becoming a member of a family. Most employees are hired at young ages and remain with the same companies throughout their working lives.

The studies of Page, Damon, and Moellering may be pertinent as well. They reported physical examinations, blood-cholesterol and uric-acid measurements, and electrocardiograms on the native population of several of the Solomon Islands and found no evidence of hypertension or coronary heart disease. They stated that, despite Western influence and adoption by some of the Western diets and religious practices, "social and family roles had remained essentially unchanged.[66]

Cassel, Patrick and Jenkins have found evidence that incongruity between a person's cultural norms—that is, the attitudes and values that he grew up with—and the social setting in which he lives and works may contribute to ill health of many sorts, including ischemic heart disease.[67] Ischemic heart disease has begun to increase to an alarming degree in Yemenite Jews who have immigrated to Israel[7] and in Ceylonese.[68] In both these populations social mores are changing rapidly, especially with regard to the emancipation of women and the acceptance of the materialistic values of Western culture.

Critique

When rigorously verifiable experimental data are not available, one must rely on carefully gathered prospective observational data. On many occasions throughout history shrewd observations have been the seeds of the growth and flowering of science. The use of prediction to validate an inference from observations, a common practice among astronomers, was found to be a useful strategy in the study reported in this book.

The data obtained over a span of twenty years in the Italian-American community of Roseto, when compared with those of neighboring communities, strongly suggest that cultural characteristics—the qualities of a social organization—affect in some way individual susceptibility to myocardial infarction and sudden death. The implication is that an emotionally supportive social environment is protective and that, by contrast, the absence of family and community support and the lack of a well-defined role in society are risk factors.

The social transition undergone by the Rosetans summarized in table 6.5 was rapid, but by no means unique. Thanks to their innate cohesiveness and the salutary influence of Father de Nisco, the Rosetans established their town on shared values and aspirations for, and willingness to, sacrifice for their progeny. Fifty years after Father de Nisco's death, a shift in social focus and aspiration from progeny to self had taken place. Mutual sharing, once typical of Roseto, gave way to competition. The formerly evident community pride and group morale were partially displaced by concerns with personal status and power. The number of three-generation households diminished, and for the first time, elderly Rosetans previously cared for at home have increasingly, since 1970, been entered into nursing homes.

TABLE 6.5
Periods of Social Change

1882-1897	Initial period of immigrant helplessness, lawlessness, conflicts, severe hardships, and exploitation by quarry owners; ended by the arrival of Father de Nisco and his appointment as parish priest
1897-1912	Period of consolidation, development of morale as a community, capped by achievement of incorporation as an independent borough
1912-1935	Evolving social change with gradual acculturation marked by emphasis on education, local self-sufficiency, and emerging political power
1935-1965	Concern with prosperity and community power; rapidly increasing acculturation, with fading of discrimination but continued strong identification with Italy (i.e., in 1962 the fiftieth anniversary of incorporation)
1965-1975	Accelerated social change as a new generation grows up in relative affluence, remote from the hardships, and discrimination endured by their forebears; young people finding careers elsewhere; sharp decline of local businesses; collapse of the taboo against ostentation
1975-1985	Continued loosening of family and community ties; competition replacing cohesion

During the early days of the twentieth century the social structure of Bangor and many other parts of rural America was similarly cohesive.

The German, French, and Scotch-Irish who inhabited the tiny villages that were absorbed into Bangor kept pretty much to themselves. When Bangor was incorporated in 1873, it was primarily an agricultural community made up of Welsh settlers and, like Roseto, its inhabitants shared the attitudes and traditions of European villagers. Over a prolonged period, spreading from east to west, America itself underwent a social transition from agrarian village life to that of an industrial nation. Those more gradual changes may not have been different from what occurred over such a comparatively short time in Roseto. The early settlers in America were villagers; the major political unit was the county, and most trade was contained within it. Neighbors helped one another, and the family and the church were the bulwarks of society. After a century, the social focus had shifted from family and community interdependence to the needs, desires, aspirations, and expectations (which ultimately became identified as rights) of individuals. Somehow, however, the individuals seemed less confident, less composed. The disquiet was evident in the comments made by Rosetans during the 1985 interviews with families at home. Typical were comments of a 25-year-old policeman whose father, owner of a construction company, had died recently of myocardial infarction at the age of 50. He described the relatively relaxed behavior of his grandparents in contrast to the fast pace of his father's and his generation. Asked why, he replied: "Different life-style; the ways... they have changed. My grandparents—the old Italian families are different from our Italian family...my wife and my children, much different. We move so much faster and we let too many things bother us." When asked, "What did they have that you don't have?" he answered; "I don't know. They had the same pressures" "Do you feel stress?", he was asked, "I try to learn from the mistakes of other people." he said "I have already had an ulcer—peptic ulcer. They say my blood pressure is too high for someone 25 years old. I feel strain—yeh—I can't compare it to what their strain is."

The increase in morbidity and mortality from coronary heart disease in the United States accompanied a shift in social values, as it did in Bangor and later, most strikingly, in Roseto. The rates began to climb steeply following the great depression and the ensuing accentuation of the importance of the individual. The trend was reinforced by developments in the intellectual world, including the emergence of Freudian and behavioral psychology and medical developments exemplified by the popular books of Dr. Benjamin Spock who prescribed new ways of bringing up children, placing the emphasis on self expression, self reliance and individual freedom.

Thus, over a period of three quarters of a century, there occurred a rise in coronary disease in America that coincided with a loosening of family cohesion and a diminished reliance on religion, together with increased emphasis on individual freedom, self-reliance and self-fulfillment. People became more competitive, more litigious and less concerned with the welfare of others. Not only was there a decline in the influence of churches and teachers, but of parents as well. By the late 1960s, the urgency of free self-expression had all but crowded out deference and considerateness and, in some quarters, even civility.

This period of social confusion marked the peak in coronary mortality in the United States. Since then, although much of the changed personal philosophy has persisted, there seems to have been a drop in heart attacks. From our observation, these radical social changes had been conspicuously delayed in Roseto, but during the late 1960s they were taking place at an accelerated rate; a sharp rise in coronary mortality occurred and continued for a few years in the face of the national decline. The rise in Roseto's coronary disease may be related not only to the nature of the social change but to its rapidity as well, that is, to the effect of change itself.

7

Predictive Significance of Various Clinical and Behavioral Measures

The two previous chapters have dealt with the correlation of social change and the prevalence of and mortality from coronary artery disease in Roseto. This chapter focuses more sharply on the influence of individual behaviors, including some generally accepted "risk factors" on outcome in terms of coronary heart disease.

Behavior Changes between 1962–63 and 1985

Diet

In the 1962–63 survey each participant was questioned concerning cooking practices and consumption of various food items as well as beer, wine, distilled spirits, and smoking. Confirmation of the dietary data was sought by visiting local food stores, where the actual patterns of purchasing were verified. Beyond that, the dieticians obtained permission from several families to observe them at mealtime. Samples corresponding to the actual amount of each food eaten by individuals were collected, placed in a metabolic bomb, and analyzed for caloric content as described elsewhere.[69] Three senior dieticians and eight student dieticians participated in the study, from which an M.A. thesis eventually evolved.[70] The investigation found that stronger than the correlation between the nature of the diet and coronary disease was the subject's habit of making major shifts in eating habits during emotional stress. In another ten-year prospective study of patients who had sustained a well-documented myocardial infarction together with matched controls, the tendency to eat either more or less when anxious or depressed was found to be highly predictive of myocardial infarction.[70]

FIGURE 7.1
Cooking and Eating Habits in Roseto

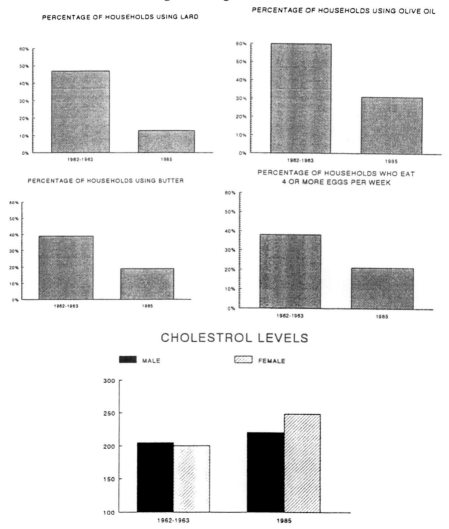

The dietary data from 1962–63 questionnaires were compared to those obtained from the 1985 follow-up examination. As reported in chapter 4, 283 Rosetans (118 men and 165 women,) who had participated in the 1962–63 survey were still alive and attended the 1985 clinic survey. In addition, 64 participants (25 men and 39 women) in the first survey who were close relatives of Rosetans living in Bangor's Fourth Ward and 122 other relatives (63 men and 59 women) living elsewhere also attended in 1985.

Despite the increased prevalence and accelerated death rate from coronary artery disease, documented in chapter 5, there had been a striking reduction in the consumption of fats and oils by Rosetans during the interval between surveys. Like the rest of the U.S. population, having been more or less continuously exposed to publicity about the dangers of fat and cholesterol, the Rosetans changed their eating habits toward what the American Heart Association called a "prudent diet," containing less lard, less butter, and fewer eggs. During the early 1960s consumption of both lard and olive oil was greater among Rosetans than Bangorians. In 1963, 47 percent of the Roseto families used lard and 57 percent used olive oil in their cooking while in Bangor 16 percent used lard and 11 percent used olive oil. By 1985 Roseto's consumption of lard had declined to 13 percent and of olive oil to 32 percent. Even corn oil and butter were being used more sparingly in cooking, and Rosetans were also consuming less butter and fewer eggs at mealtime (figure 7.1). Despite their reduced consumption of animal fats, there occurred a slight increase in the mean serum concentration of cholesterol among Rosetans.

Exercise

The case for physical exercise in the primary prevention of coronary heart disease has been reviewed by the U.S. Preventive Services Task Force.[71] While it is difficult to quantify physical activity or inactivity, the available evidence finds nearly a two-fold risk of coronary artery disease in relatively sedentary people. Just how much exercise is required to reduce the risk has not been determined, but the task force report indicates that regular, sustained low-level exercise, such as walking, may be more protective than the more strenuous aerobic exercise aimed at cardiorespiratory fitness. The vast experience of Cooper's aerobic research group in Dallas has been recently summarized by Gordon and Scott.[72] From

TABLE 7.1
NUMBER OF DEAD WITH CHOLESTEROL UNDER 200

	AGE		Hypertension	DIAST 90+	Diab	% OF SUBJECTS MORE THAN 15 LBS. OVERWEIGHT
	<65	65+				
Men	11	6	2	7	2	41.2%
Control	11	6	2	7	0	5.9%
Women	7	4	2	2	0	36.4%
Control	10	1	3	2	1	36.4%

NUMBER OF DEAD WITH CHOLESTEROL OVER 200

	<65	65+	Hypertension	DIAST 90+	Diab	OVERWEIGHT
Men	40	7	5	24	1	36.2%
Control	41	6	3	16	0	36.2%
Women	16	6	7	13	0	50%
Control	16	6	1	12	0	27.3%

Cholesterol Levels	No. of People	Totals			Male			Female	
		Died	Survived	Total	Died	Survived	Total	Died	Survived
Under 200	565	28	18	253	17	11	312	11	7
200–249	305	46	14	157	31	7	148	15	7
250–275	67	12	4	38	8	2	29	4	2
276–300	27	5	2	15	3	2	12	2	0
301–325	19	1	0	6	0	0	13	1	0
326–400	34	2	1	20	2	1	14	0	0
Over 400	27	3	1	16	3	1	11	0	0

their work and that of others, it appears to be well established that a consistent habit of moderate physical exercise is significantly protective against coronary artery disease and sudden death.

Whether exercise played a salutary role among Rosetans during the early years, and, conversely whether reduced exercise may have been harmful during recent decades is difficult to assess. It is clear, however, that the majority of Rosetan men were engaged in strenuous exercise in the slate quarries for at least the first fifty years of Roseto's existence and that substantially fewer have been so active during the past fifty years. Also, as already pointed out, there is much less walking about in Roseto than before. Thus a decrease in physical activity has been clearly evident over the span of years between the two surveys.

Smoking

In 1962-1963, 32 percent of Roseto men and 12 percent of Roseto women smoked cigarettes. By 1985 smoking had decreased to 22 percent among men and 9 percent among women. The average number of years since having quit was nine for women and seven for men. The number of cigarette smokers in Bangor was 35 percent among men and 16 percent among women in 1964. The figures for 1985 in Bangor were not ascertained.

Alcohol

Among the changes in social behavior in Roseto was a decline in the practice of wine making, coupled with an accompanying decline in the consumption of wine. Nearly half the households made their own wine in 1963; by 1985 only 10 percent, mainly the elderly, were making wine. The consumption of distilled spirits and beer changed very little between surveys except that more women were consuming whiskey, brandy, and beer in 1985.

Predictors

Most epidemiological studies have explored the relevance of risk factors and other purported indicators of susceptibility to myocardial infarction or sudden death by comparing prevalence or incidence of a disorder in large groups of people. Less frequent have been prospective studies focused on individual subjects before and after exposure to a purported hazard. In our case the presumed hazard is the rapid renunciation of long-observed social values and behavior, the manifestations of which were few and very slowly progressive until approximately 1965, when evidence of such a social change became conspicuous.

Predictive Significance of Generally Accepted Risk Factors

Cholesterol Concentration

The relevance of the serum concentration of cholesterol and its protein vectors to the pathogenesis of coronary atherosclerosis and to complications and consequences therefrom, including myocardial infarction and sudden death, has been assiduously explored and reported on in a vast accumulation of medical literature. In 1990 Pekkanen and colleagues studied 10-year mortality in more than 2,500 white men 40 to 69 years of age, 17 percent of whom had signs of cardiovascular disease at the start of the study.[73] They found a more than doubling of death from cardiovascular disease in individuals with no evidence of it at the start of the study whose initial serum cholesterol level was above 240, as compared with those whose levels were less than 239.

Among Rosetans and their family members who participated in the 1962–63 survey in Roseto, cholesterol data were available on 507 men and 539 women. Among that group, 64 men and 33 women died of myocardial infarction between 1964 and 1990, and 24 men and 16 women experienced a well-documented myocardial infarction during the interval but recovered.

Figure 7.2 displays the percentage of fatal myocardial infarctions and infarctions with survival over a span of 27 years in seven ranges of serum cholesterol concentration measured in 1962–63. The serum cholesterol was less than 200 mg/dl in more than half the subjects. Myocardial infarction with or without fatality occurred among 7 percent of that group and 19 percent of those whose cholesterol was over 200. Subjects whose serum concentration exceeded 200 mg/dl were more likely to die of myocardial infarction during the next twenty-seven years than those with cholesterols below 200 (P <0.01). The risk of myocardial infarction increased with higher ranges up to 300. After that the numbers were too

FIGURE 7.2
Percentage of Recoveries and Deaths from Myocardial Infarctions

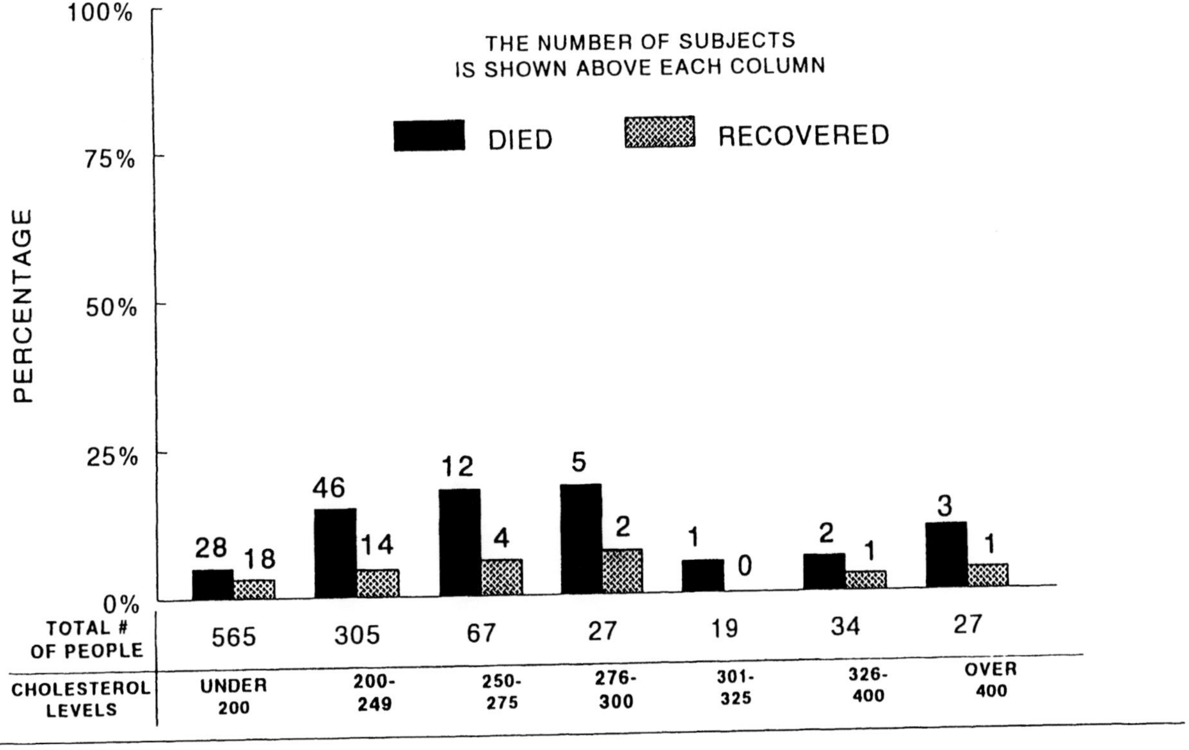
100%
75%
50%
25%
0%
PERCENTAGE
THE NUMBER OF SUBJECTS
IS SHOWN ABOVE EACH COLUMN
DIED
RECOVERED
28
18
46
14
12
4
5
2
1
0
2
1
3
1
TOTAL #
OF PEOPLE
565
305
67
27
19
34
27
CHOLESTEROL
LEVELS
UNDER
200
200-
249
250-
275
276-
300
301-
325
326-
400
OVER
400

small for analysis. Fewer than 20 percent of the subjects with values above 200 experienced myocardial infarction during the 22 year span.

A similar analysis was made on the same sample with respect to hypertension identified by a history of treated hypertension, or by a blood pressure measurement of 140/95 or greater during the physical examination. Evidence of diabetes and obesity were included in the analysis, the latter being defined as weighing more than 20 pounds above ideal weight in relation to age and height. Those who died of myocardial infarction and those who had experienced MI and survived were compared to controls who had neither died nor experienced myocardial infarction. The controls were matched to the subjects on age, sex, and cholesterol level (Table 7.1). Although there was more hypertension and obesity among those decedents and the recoverers whose cholesterol was 200 or above, no statistically significant differences were established between patients and controls. Among those individuals whose serum cholesterol in 1962–63 was below 200, the complications of hypertension, diabetes, and obesity were infrequent among both decedents and controls.

This suggestive finding fits well with current views of the contribution of cholesterol to coronary disease. A striking finding was that obesity was much more prominent among men with cholesterol values below 200 who died of myocardial infarction than among their controls, while obesity was more prominent among women whose cholesterol concentration was 200 and above than among their controls.

Oxidized Cholesterol

Despite the widespread alarm among cardiologists and the general public concerning saturated fat and cholesterol in the diet, the case against cholesterol in natural foods such as milk and eggs has still to be firmly established. In fact, there is substantial evidence that oxidized cholesterol, not the pure cholesterol in fresh eggs and dairy products has been responsible for many of the atherosclerotic lesions in experimental studies involving cholesterol feeding of animals.

In 1976 Imai, Taylor and Werthessen showed that atherosclerotic lesions cannot be produced in rabbits by feeding pure cholesterol but can be produced by USP cholesterol which, when left at room temperature, becomes oxidized.[74] Later, Imai repeated the experiment in pigs, and showed that USP cholesterol feeding produced "extensive medial and intimal necrosis and arterial smooth muscle cell death followed by repair with fibromuscular thickening" Feeding pure cholesterol produced no tissue change.[75]

Palinski and associates showed that the LDL fraction of lipoproteins is susceptible to oxidation in vivo,[76] suggesting that in order for circulating cholesterol to be involved in atherogenesis, it may be necessary for the LDL to become oxidized. Also relevant to atherosclerosis is the demonstration by Mitchinson and associates that oxidized LDL is stored in macrophages to produce the characteristic sequestration of foam cells in the arterial wall.[77]

During a conference on the pathogenic significance of pure vs. oxidized cholesterol sponsored in 1977 by the Office of Naval Research, Leland Smith observed that pure cholesterol has no odor but, when left exposed at room temperature within a few days, develops an odor as autoxidation begins before it can be detected chemically.[75]

Bruce Taylor reported studies of the Masai in East Africa whose chief article of diet is cow's milk mixed with cow's blood. He reported that the Masai maintain a serum cholesterol concentration of 135 mg/dl throughout old age and have very little arteriosclerosis.[79] Additionally it was learned that cholesterol made inside the body of a mammal is protected by natural antioxidants.

Taylor suggested the possibility that fluctuations in arterial morbidity in the United States may have been influenced by methods of food preservation as well as shelf life and changes during transportation.

Earlier studies of the angiotoxicity of peroxidation were published by George Mann in 1974.[80] He and his colleagues focused initially on the small blood vessel lesions of diabetes. Later Verlangiere and Sestito showed that insulin promotes the uptake of the antioxidant ascorbic acid in coronary endothelium.[81]

Polyunsaturated fats are, of course, the lipids that are most susceptible to oxidation by free radicals. Chicken has been recommended by heart conscious dieticians as a substitute for meats containing more saturated fat but Pikul and Kummerow found that chicken meat begins accumulating oxidized lipids within 24 hours of cooking—even though the meat had been refrigerated immediately after cooking.[82] Free oxygen and hydroxyl radicals are generally harmful to lipid membranes throughout the body by impairing their ability to keep out calcium. Ischemia has been shown to stimulate the production of free radicals in human tissue, including the heart and also to impair the activity of natural antioxidants in the body.[83]

It is of special interest that the oxidized cholesterol molecule, 25-hydroxycholesterol, is not only destructive to endothelial cells but, as normally present in low concentration in blood serum, also acts as a natural inhibitor of cholesterol synthesis in the liver.[84] This suggests that further investigations of the well known ability of polyunsaturated fats to lower serum cholesterol should examine the possibility of oxidation of the polyunsaturates due to time and exposure.

Variability in Cholesterol Concentration

Although not usually emphasized, it has been known for several years that, independent of diet, the serum concentration of cholesterol normally varies from time to time during a day, and from day to day as well. Wide swings in cholesterol concentration associated with stressful life experiences have been reported in subjects maintained for weeks or months on a fixed diet.[85]

Following the early work of Groen and colleagues,[86] several workers have studied the serum concentration of cholesterol and lipids in people under stress (for example, students before, during, and after examinations). All of them, including Thomas and Murphy,[87] Wertlake et al.[88] Grundy and Griffin,[89] and Dreyfuss and Czackes[90] found higher values of cholesterol during the stressful periods than otherwise. Dreyfuss also measured the clotting time and found it accelerated in thirty-six medical students on the morning of a final examination in medicine. Rahe and colleagues made similar observations during training of Naval underwater demolition teams.[91] In other studies reported by Groover,[92] Friedman, Rosenmann,[93] and Hammersten et al.[94] there was evidence that the responses of lipid regulating mechanisms occur in association with personality characteristics and behavior.

Other Indicators

Perturbations of several homeostatic regulatory mechanisms other than those that control cholesterol concentration have been found to correlate with emotionally stressful life experiences and also to be predictive of myocardial infarction or sudden death. Among them is reduced periodic heart rate variability or sinus arrhythmia.[95] Wenckebach and Winterberg in 1927 recognized sinus arrhythmia as a sign of a healthy heart,[96] and his pupil, Sherf, and Boyd considered a perfectly regular heart beat to be a suspicious sign of heart disease.[97] Later, Gross reported that the amplitude of periodic heart rate variability was reduced in association with angina pectoris.[98]

In 1971 Wolf observed that the range of heart rate variability in individuals who had suffered a myocardial infarction months or years in the past was reduced and much narrower than the range in healthy control subjects of comparable age, even though the exercise tolerance of the coronary patients, as tested on a treadmill, might equal or exceed that of their individually matched control.[99] Moreover, the degree of damping of heart rate variability among these subjects appeared to have prognostic significance with respect to recurrent myocardial infarction or sudden death. The reduced amplitude of sinus arrhythmia known to accompany aging persists during sleep, but the apparent "reining in" of rhythmic heart rate variability in coronary patients may be lost during sleep. In fact, the swings of sinus arrhythmia may even be exaggerated. Long ignored by cardiologists, reduced periodic heart rate variability has now been confirmed as an ominous sign, but the recent reports have failed to acknowledge the original work.[100,101]

In other areas exaggerated variability may occur, as shown by Schneider and Costiloe, who found increased variability of heart rate to startle in the patients with coronary artery disease.[102] Hampton and colleagues, studying variability in the mechanisms that regulate blood clotting, found increased variability in plasma concentration of fibrinogen and silicone clotting time among patients with coronary heart disease as compared to matched controls; they further observed that such variability is predictive of sudden death in patients who have sustained a myocardial infarction.[103] Recently their findings have been confirmed.[104]

Among electrocardiographic predictors of sudden death are prolongation of the QT interval, which contains the period of repolarization of the ventricles.[105] Such prolongation may precede a series of premature ventricular beats, another ominous harbinger of sudden death. Such a sequence has been shown to be triggered by emotionally stressful circumstances.[106] In keeping with an hypothesis that the duration of QT is related to the force of ventricular contraction,[107] the ballistocardiographic measurement of the force of ventricular contraction was found to be predictive of sudden death in patients who have recovered from a well-documented myocardial infarction.[108]

There is a good deal of evidence that instability or lability of neurophysiological regulatory mechanisms precedes clinical disorders of various sorts and that the degree of lability may be of prognostic significance[109] Sixty-seven male and female subjects who had sustained a well-documented myocardial infarction, matched with controls according to age, sex, height, weight, educational background, and type of job, were studied prospectively over a period of ten years. At periodic visits every four to six weeks, measurements of a variety of physiological and psychological indicators were made, including (1) dietary behavior, (2) serum cholesterol and uric acid concentration, (3) blood clotting factors,[103] (4) treadmill performance (EKG), (5) ballistocardiographic data, (6) coronary blood flow, measured by a radioisotopic technic[110] (7) heart rate and BP responses to startle; and (8) indicators of personality adjustment, (9) social satisfaction, and (10) depression. All the observations were made independently by members of a collaborating group.[111] At the end of four years each investigator was asked to predict on the basis of his or her measurements which of the patients or controls was at the greatest risk of recurrent myocardial infarction or sudden death. Of the thirty-one patients who died suddenly or of definitely established myocardial infarction (nine of the thirty-one were not autopsied), all but two were on two or more of the lists. So were two subjects who committed suicide and eight who suffered no recurrent infarct. Among the control group there were one correct and five false positive predictions.

Highly statistically significant predictions were made by the dietary data, which had reflected major change in food consumption accompanying emotional swings.[70] Lability in blood clotting measures and the ballistocardiographic pattern also ranked high as predictors.[108] Less striking, but significantly predictive were coronary blood flow monitoring and lability of the response to startle.[112] Psychological factors, especially the joyless striving of the Sisyphus pattern which closely resembled the Type A behavior of Friedman and Rosenman[8] were also shown to have prognostic significance.[114]

Considering the consequences and predictive significance of lability in the central neuroregulatory systems that ultimately control all aspects of metabolic balance and the behavior of the heart, blood vessels, and other tissues, all environmental forces that may disturb the homeostatic systems, including social and psychologically significant circumstances in the lives of individuals, must be taken into account. As Bruhn has pointed out, however: "individual variability is often obscured through the common use of group means [which] may mask important differences in physiological measurements taken over time."[115]

As important as behaviors such as diet or smoking appear to be from studies of large groups of more-or-less anonymous individuals, they have not been of significant predictive value over a twenty-five year span of time in Roseto. On the other hand, attention directed to broader aspects of behavior of individuals and groups, specifically those that lead to or reflect social disintegration, has suggested a strong influence of individual social values and collective morale on the heart and coronary vessels. The loss of social stability, as reflected in the loosening of family ties and the weakening of community cohesion, appear from the 1985 sociological interviews to have induced a sense of uncertainty about the future among Rosetans, with a variety of accompanying apprehensions and emotional conflicts and perhaps undue variability in vital homeostatic systems.

8

Social Change 1963–1988

The structured sociological interviews conducted in Roseto and Bangor in the 1960s and 1980s served as a source of information on social change from the viewpoint of the inhabitants of each town. These data were supplemented from the careful studies of Valletta[32] and Bianco[34] and from documents made available by officials and organizations of the two towns.

Shortly before the turn of the century, Italian settlements had appeared in several parts of Pennsylvania, each with settlers from a different region of Italy. Only Roseto, however, became a community exclusively owned and operated by Italians. Most of the inhabitants had emigrated from a town of the same name near the Adriatic coast, Roseto Val Fortore. The Italians in West Bangor, less than three miles from Roseto, originated mainly from Sorrento and other towns near Naples. Those who settled in nearby Pen Argyl had come chiefly from the northeastern region of Italy close to Venice. There was vigorous rivalry among the three Italian communities during the early years in America, but also a certain amount of intermarriage.

Education

With the influence of Father de Nisco, who had arrived fourteen years after the original immigration, Roseto gained an advantage over the other Italian communities. Subsequent incorporation as an independent bor-

The collaboration of Judith Lasker and Brenda Egolf was indispensable in the development of this chapter, especially with respect to the quantified data on social change.

ough further boosted Roseto's prestige among other Italian immigrants in the region. One of Father de Nisco's prime objectives was to provide education for the young. The first formal schooling in Roseto took place in the home of a priest, Rev. Antonio Cerutti. His efforts were soon supplemented by classes held in two small one room school houses. After incorporation in 1912 the energetic Rosetans lost no time in obtaining a public school. Five Rosetans were appointed by the county court as the board of directors. The building of Columbus School, grades 1-8, was completed in 1913. Four young Roseto women were qualified as initial faculty. Later, a few teachers were recruited from nearby towns. There was no high school.

By 1940 less than 10 percent of Rosetans had had more than a grammar school education, while 40 percent of Bangorians had experienced some high school or college (fig. 8.1). That year the Rev. Joseph Ducci, pastor of the church of Our Lady of Mt. Carmel, succeeded in attracting a group of Salesian nuns to Roseto from New Jersey to establish a convent. By 1945 the nuns had started a kindergarten and primary classes. Two years later a building for the parochial school was completed, and by 1951 Pius X High School was established in Roseto across the street from Our Lady of Mt. Carmel. Italians from other communities began sending their children to Pius X, and soon the student body included catholics from other ethnic groups in surrounding communities.

Marriage

The school contributed to gradual social change in Roseto as new generations gained more education than their parents and grandparents and as the young people came in contact with non-Rosetans during the school day. The first social tradition to change was the selection of marriage partners. For more than thirty years after the original immigration, nearly all Rosetans married within their community, and usually within their religious denomination. There was, however, much less social disapproval of interdenominational marriages by Rosetans to Rosetans than of marriages outside the community, even to Roman Catholics.

During the decade 1935-1944 more than 93 percent of the spouses were Italian. This pattern held pretty well until World War II, but after

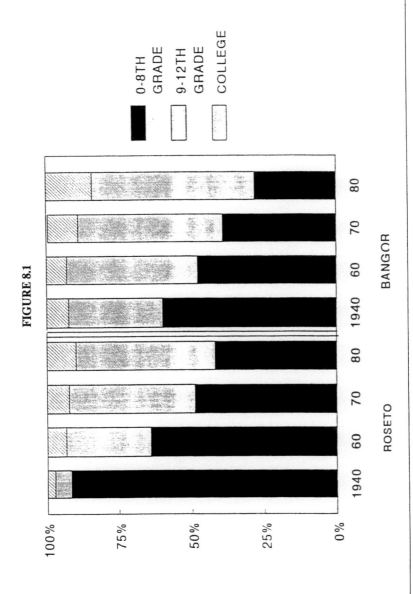

FIGURE 8.1

Percentage of Inhabitants at Each Educational Level

the influx of young people into Pius X and the experience of World War II, the marriage records show that about 30 percent of new spouses were only half-Italian, and a few were non-Italian. After marriage a good many of the mixed couples moved to other communities, especially Bangor, since marrying non-Italians was still mildly disapproved of. When Rosetans married Italians from nearby communities, most of the brides moved to their husband's town where, in the case of Roseto, a few years had to pass before the new spouse was fully accepted. The reluctance to accept non-Rosetans and non-Italians in Roseto cooled gradually, so that by 1985 when approximately 80 percent of Rosetans were marrying non-Italians, the prejudice was all but gone (fig. 8.2).

We were able to obtain information on interdenominational marriages performed at Our Lady of Mt. Carmel by studying the church marriage records, which had been meticulously maintained since 1925. The church performed an average of twenty-four marriages per year. During the decade 1925-1934, 87 percent of the marriages were between two Catholic partners. In subsequent decades that figure declined slowly but progressively, until the 1965-1974 decade saw the percentage of Catholic to Catholic fall sharply from 75.5 percent to 58.3 percent. By 1984 the percentage was down to 52.2.

At the time of the 1962-63 survey nearly all new spouses had at least one Italian parent, usually a Rosetan. Many of the new non-Roseto spouses did not participate in the surveys, although their Rosetan partners may have done so. The children of the 1945 spurt in marriages to non-Rosetans who were non-Italian or had only one Italian parent were too young to have participated in the 1962-1963 survey, but they did constitute eleven of the 364 Rosetans who took part in the second survey.

Employment and Income

The sophisticating influences of education and marriage outside the community also affected the business life of Roseto, at first accelerating local industry and later inhibiting it as the business men became involved in regional industry and developed out-of-town social connections.

When we studied Roseto and Bangor in the early 1960s, nearly 70 percent of Rosetans were unskilled or semiskilled workmen, while fewer than 60 percent of Bangorians were in that category. By 1980 the percentage of the unskilled or semiskilled in Roseto had fallen to near

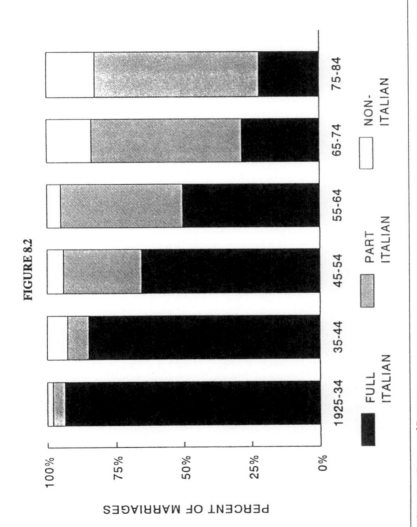

FIGURE 8.2

Ethnic Identity of Marriage Partners of Rosetans

50 percent, below that of Bangor, while by that time 20 percent of Rosetans, but only 15 percent of Bangorians had reached the proprietor or professional categories (fig. 8.3). By 1962 Roseto had produced twelve physicians and dentists, only one of whom practiced in Roseto, seven in Bangor, three elsewhere in eastern Pennsylvania, and one was in New Jersey; of the six Rosetans who had become lawyers, none were practicing in Roseto. Four lawyers were in Bangor and two were in California. Not surprisingly, the annual income of Roseto increased in relation to Bangor, going from approximately 60 percent of that of Bangor in 1940 to more than 90 percent in 1980 (fig. 8.4).

Local Businesses

Many enterprising Rosetans, some of whom still held their jobs in the slate quarries, maintained small businesses in their homes. Prior to World War II virtually all shopping was done locally. There were three or more baker, butcher, and barber shops and a dozen grocery stores. There were four photographers, two jewelers, five tailors, half a dozen pool parlors and three theaters. There were also two cigar makers, a cheese factory, three hotels with bars, four plumbing and hardware companies, and five restaurants. Most of the shops and businesses occupied the ground floor or basement of the owners' homes.

In 1905 a new opportunity for employment arrived when the New York firm of S. Liebovitz induced the residents of Roseto to establish textile finishing factories to help replace the outlawed New York sweat shops, which had employed underage children. Those Rosetans who invested became proprietors and entrepreneurs. Some of the Rosetans working in the slate quarry took on the mechanical tasks in the textile factories, but most of the machine operators were mainly women for whom the nearby "blouse mills" provided a way to supplement their family's income.

By the 1950s more organized businesses had appeared in Roseto including a nonferrous foundry and a paper-box company, but mainly more textile mills. In 1962 there were sixteen of them employing more than 450 workers. They engaged mainly in making ladies' blouses for the New York market. That year a prosperous Roseto celebrated its Golden Jubilee, the fiftieth anniversary of its incorporation, which was attended by the Italian ambassador and the local congressman.

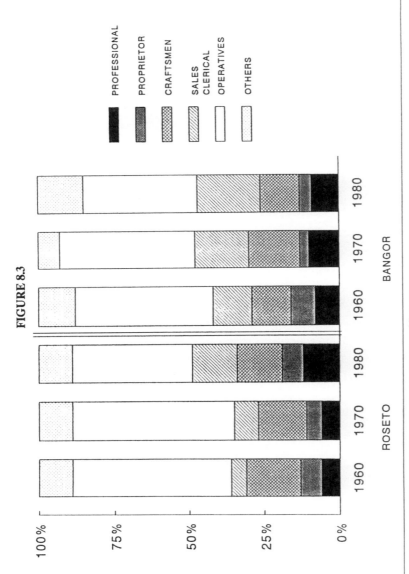

FIGURE 8.3

PROFESSIONAL
PROPRIETOR
CRAFTSMEN
SALES CLERICAL
OPERATIVES
OTHERS

ROSETO

1960 1970 1980

BANGOR

1960 1970 1980

100% 75% 50% 25% 0%

Percentage of Residents in Different Job Classifications in Roseto and Bangor

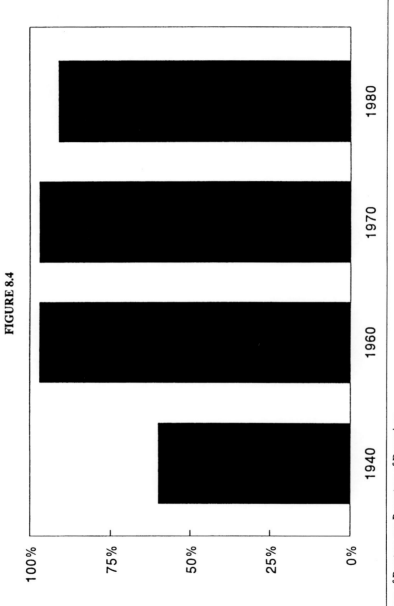

FIGURE 8.4

Income of Rosetans as a Percentage of Bangorians

Within the next decade a trend away from local concerns and toward involvement with regional and national activities accelerated. Hotels and restaurants closed and the number of shops diminished as the younger generation no longer took over the management from their aging parents and Rosetans began patronizing malls and restaurants away from Roseto. Some surveying, plumbing, landscaping, and building contractors held on, but their numbers diminished. Only the number of garages and repair shops increased.

Music

As mentioned in chapter 2, music was important to the inhabitants of Roseto Val Fortore; so it was in Roseto, Pennsylvania, as well. The music for the Golden Jubilee was supplied by the Roseto Cornet Band, which had been organized in 1895 under the baton of Philip Carrescia, who had been a member of the Brass Band of Roseto Val Fortore. A later leader was Michelangelo Donatelli, whose ancestor, Egidio Donatelli, in 1790, organized and conducted that famous orchestra, which gave concerts throughout Italy.[25] A marching Drum and Bugle Corps existed off and on from 1947 to 1960, to be revived in 1984 in time for the 1987 Diamond Jubilee of Roseto. There was also at one time a Pius X Band, a Roseto Boys Band and a few other musical groups.

Local Organizations

Like the musical groups, Roseto's social organizations, religious and otherwise, played a major part in the life of the community. There were men's and women's religious clubs for all ages, organized mainly by the communicants of the church of Our Lady of Mt. Carmel. In addition the town had spawned countless more secular groups. Twenty-five of these small organizations participated in the celebration of the Diamond Jubilee.

The Marconi Social Club was founded in 1903. Its function was primarily to promote fellowship among Italians in Roseto and nearby communities and to provide a gathering place for the men in the evening. In 1930 the club built a handsome new lodge on Garibaldi Avenue, next to what was then a hotel but later was occupied by another club, the Martocci-Capobianco American Legion Post. The Roseto Volunteer Fire

Department also maintains a meeting room and bar for its members and supporters and there are Democratic and Republican political clubs as well.

A council for the Knights of Columbus, named for Father de Nisco, was established in 1954 to include not only Rosetan Roman Catholics but those from surrounding slate-belt communities as well. A year later a ladies auxiliary was formed.

In 1918, following World War I, boy scout troops were chartered in both the Protestant and Catholic churches of Roseto. A girl scout troop followed in the mid 1930s.

The Roseto Rod and Gun Club, founded in 1939 and chartered in 1941, eventually spawned a ladies' auxiliary in 1956. Other sporting organizations included the Roseto baseball Giants, which was started by Father de Nisco in 1905 and supported by him. The baseball, basketball, and football teams flourished mainly in the 1930s and 1940s before television brought sports into the home, but organized baseball for youngsters in Roseto has continued. In 1965 a chapter of UNICO, a charitable organization aimed at community service and developing leadership among Americans of Italian descent, was formed. Its ladies' auxiliary was not established until 1978. A senior citizens' organization was begun in 1974.

Information about local clubs and organizations was obtained from church records and Roseto and Bangor historical publications as well as the sociological surveys carried out in the mid-1960s and 1980s. Overall seventy-one organized groups were identified between the two communities; thirteen of them no longer exist. Recommendations from community leaders helped us identify an informant for most organizations (some of the defunct groups had no one available for interview). A total of fifty-eight informants were interviewed: twenty-four concerning organizations in Roseto, thirty in Bangor. In the course of a semistructured interview lasting one and a half hours, the informant was asked about the history, membership, and activities of the organization and how it had changed over the past twenty years. The number of clubs and organizations in each town (twenty-four in Roseto, thirty in Bangor) demonstrates the greater density of organizational life in Roseto with a population less than a third that of Bangor. During the period of our early survey, the Roseto clubs were more active than were the Bangor clubs, and their attendance at meetings was more reliable.

The organizations were classified according to whether they were locally or nationally based. Of those located in Roseto, 62.5 percent were local, compared to Bangor organizations, of which 63.3 percent were branches of national groups. Informants from national organizations located in Roseto reported an increase in their membership during recent years whereas those in Bangor reported a decrease. Thus, while Rosetans initially formed more local groups, over time they increased their participation in those organizations that connected them to national activities and issues.

Over half of the fifteen Rosetan organizations with a national base had a rule of membership that required applicants to be Italian, to be married to an Italian, or be a relative of a member. By contrast, only a quarter of national organizations located in Bangor required that one be a relative of a member, and none had an ethnic standard for joining. Roseto organizations, especially the local ones, admitted male members only.

By 1985 the informants were complaining about a decline in interest in their organizations, particularly among the younger people. Forty percent of Roseto informants and a third of those in Bangor observed that their group was losing members.

During the thirty years of our study, there have been fifteen church organizations for youth, including such groups as the Boy Scouts, the Young Girl Choir, and Junior Holy Name. Total membership in all of these groups declined from 1,276 in 1963 to 479 in 1986. Church records also show a decline in membership from 2,716 to 2,544 and especially in the proportion of members who regularly attend mass, which in thirty years had dropped from 52 percent to 43 percent.

The Shift Toward American Values and Aspirations

While Rosetans were becoming better educated and more prosperous as their contacts with the outside world broadened, they were also becoming less family-centered and less cohesive, less willing to sacrifice for family, friends, and neighbors. As a community, they were also becoming less self-contained.

At the time of our initial survey in 1962-63, the sybaritic tendencies of the wealthy Rosetans were largely concealed. Occasionally, a few Rosetan couples would take off for Atlantic City for a weekend of spending and self-indulgence, but back in Roseto their behavior was as modest and frugal as ever. Around 1965 a few expensive automobiles began to appear on the streets. We soon learned that some of the families had joined country clubs. The occasional visits to Atlantic City were replaced by weekends in Las Vegas and luxury cruises. Not long afterward, construction of new houses began around the edges of the town, large houses, some of them ranch-type with broad, green lawns, fountains, and swimming pools. One housewife, after a year in such elegant surroundings, stated:

> I'm sorry we moved. Everything is very modern here, very nice. I have everything I need, except people. When we lived in town, the neighbors were always in my kitchen or I was in theirs. We talked. We knew what was going on, and there was always someone around to help you and to keep you from feeling lonely. I miss that, but I guess I will never go back.

Most of the abandoned houses on the main street, Garibaldi Avenue, and elsewhere in the center of town were bought by the younger generation who had been living in three-generation households. In 1960, with a population of 1,630, there were 456 houses in Roseto. By 1970, although the population had decreased to 1,538, the number of houses had increased to 477. The trend continued through 1980, at which time the population was 1,484 and the households numbered 561. Thus, as the population fell by nearly 150, the houses in Roseto increased in number by more than 100.

In 1974 Roseto was visited by a reporter, Robert Oppedisano, from the *IAM Magazine*, [30] who described the vast changes in the town and in its people:

> For years, for longer than anyone has any right to expect, Roseto, Pennsylvania, has been the purest Italian community in the United States. It sits quietly on a ridge in eastern Pennsylvania, fifteen miles north of Easton....There is a small scale to Roseto, and not due solely to the size of its population. There is a village feel, a human sense of proportion, a closeness peculiar to southern Europe. Everything is right here, on the street, with none of that peculiarly reclusive chill common to, say, New England. The streets were meant for walking, for *la passeggiata*, for talking, for gossiping, for watching each other....But there are no people on the street.

> Those expecting to find a Little-Italy-In-the-Mountains, complete with swarming children, strutting street corner men, and housewives in flower-print housedresses should be forewarned.... The talk in town is almost always about how much money there is in a town so small. There's a lot of money here, a lot, said Mrs. Matt LeDonne, who works in her husband's bakery. 'All these homes here are beautiful inside, and everybody's got two, three cars. And all the Cadillacs!' What they gave up was the protective culture of peasant Italy, apparently. What they got in return was the chance

to become Americans—rich ones, troubled ones, real ones. So run the academic explanations. Rosetans have their own.... Roseto, it seems, had met the enemy, and it was itself.... The past lingers in Roseto, where rootedness and continuity are almost mythic qualities. Life was invariably simpler, more rewarding, less troublesome, even if it was harder. The present, for all its rewards—and Roseto is a prosperous town—never fully satisfied.

People talk of an easier, less complicated life, where hard work was the only concern, and large families and many friends the major joys.... "I'd say the good years, they was from 1900 to 1914," said Phillip Capobianco, who is 84. 'Then we work hard, but not have a fast life. Now everybody competes, and they live fast, It's no good.' Mr. Capobianco worked the slate quarries 20 years before buying the Roseto Hotel in 1924. The quarries were, and are, open pits, 200 feet deep, where men slide along narrow edges to chip away chunks of rock. It is dangerous work, yet Mr. Capobianco calls that period of his life his happiest. The feeling among older Rosetans about their community is so strong that hardships vanish from memory....Mr. Capobianco sold his hotel to a Mr. Ron Striba, a musician from nearby Pen Argyl who operated it as a bar and restaurant....The old hotel had been the heart of Roseto; once it shook with the sounds of dances, weddings and feasts. Most of the time, though, it was a place where men could sit, drink wine, play *tresette* or *scopa* and smoke black Toscano cigars....

The first thing Ron Striba did was raise the price of beer to twenty cents a glass. It used to be a dime. 'I had to do it,' he said. 'When I took over here two years ago, the old timers would come in and sit all day with one glass of wine, and I'd maybe make a buck. When I raised the price, they complained. Can you believe it? They had rolls of hundreds in their pockets, but kept their fingers on the change.' ...Ron Striba told his plans. He was starting small. 'Now I've got Evonne, my go-go dancer. She's 40 with 5 kids and not a stretch mark. You believe it? We've got 60, 70 guys here every Saturday night with scarlet fever. This place moves!' Down at the other end, Louis Trigiani, Jr., just out of East Stroudsburg State College, was complaining. "There's no action here. I mean all anybody ever thinks about is food. Food and Cadillacs."

Writing at about the time of the rapid social change occurring in Roseto, Marvin Sussman called attention to what he saw as a widespread social trend in America in his article "Personal Happiness as an Emerging Ethic." "The essence of the personal happiness value," he wrote, "is that self-fulfillment is a continuing quest and that extensive self denial or sacrifice is unnecessary."[116]

Home interviews conducted in 1986 with members of Roseto families had yielded messages that were strikingly similar with each generation, but sharply contrasting from generation to generation. In one large family that occupied three adjoining houses in the center of Roseto, the reply to a question about change in the community by the 88-year-old grandmother was, "Big, big change, big change! Too much freedom—the girls and the boys. Too much freedom! I no like; I'm old fashioned." Her

62-year- old daughter, whose husband had died of myocardial infarction at 50 years of age in 1971 and whose son was in medical school, spoke of the new educational opportunities, adding, "Aren't all mothers that have their sons becoming doctors proud? I am very proud of him." Her 40-year-old son, who had married an Irish Catholic from Boston, spoke of two-car families: "We never had a two-car family. We are very aggressive to get another job or to earn more money to attain a two-car family." Commenting on the new homes built on the edges of Roseto, he said, "The homes are well back from the main artery. They want to display their front yards. They want to show people what they have done and what they have."

Finally, his 22-year-old daughter, married to the son of a developer of German ancestry, said, "I envy other people. I work hard so what I do have I am proud of and I hope to be able to have more things. I worry about it—I'll be honest."

This vivid contrast in expression from four generations of Rosetans could probably be identified in most American families, but starting two or three generations earlier. The implications, of course, go beyond the family to the community itself. Implicitly the achievement of community solidarity and pride demands work, personal sacrifice and concern for others.

To characterize properly the state of fulfillment of a community or of a person living there requires attention to qualitative, not just quantitative data. An attempt to quantify personal satisfaction or group morale would be uninformative, even frivolous. As Angus Campbell put it: "Can it be said that the satisfaction of a college student who has been elected captain of his football team is equal to that of a candidate who has been elected to the Senate?.... the satisfactions are equal in the sense that two bottles may be equally full, even if one holds much more than the other."

During the early 1980s several completely non-Italian families took up residence in Roseto. To the "old timers" this meant that the town's integrity had been violated or compromised by dilution with "outsiders." Nevertheless, during the transition, there were no efforts to bolster the unity of the town. The Roseto families failed to provide support for the integrating resources in the community such as restaurants, taverns, stores, and social clubs. As previously mentioned, even the attendance at church and involvement in church organizations slackened. Many Rosetans were now finding social life, entertainment, diversion and companionship outside of town. Fewer households contained more than one or two generations. Some of the families had even discontinued their traditional annual or semiannual reunion.

Some of the more cohesive families strove to stem the tide but found that, in addition to the temptations of the consumer society around them, there appeared to be aspects of the traditional Italian domestic life that encouraged rebellion. When a 92-year-old woman, who had been born in Roseto, was asked why her five daughters had chosen non-Italian husbands, she replied with a short account of her own life. Still a charming, friendly, lighthearted woman at 92, she said that as a teenager she had been very popular with the young men in Roseto and had agreed to marry one of them, whom she "loved very much." Her parents, however, had selected another of her suiters, a recent Italian immigrant who had a job in a slate quarry and whom her parents declared was a "hard worker who will take good care of you." He turned out to be domineering and demanding. The bride had wanted to have only two or three children but her husband insisted on a large family. She eventually bore twelve children, ten of whom survived childhood. "Do you understand," she asked, "why my daughters married non-italian men?" When the boys were 5 to 10 years old, her husband required them to work in the garden and orchard throughout the summer and to cut wood during the winter. Four of the boys who had married Italian girls eventually divorced and remarried non-Italian women. Not all older-generation husbands were so patriarchal. There were matriarchs in Roseto, too, but there was evidence that, in an age when parental authority was being questioned throughout America, the young in Roseto were restive in their traditional family structure.

Regardless of whether rebellion against the traditional authority of the older generation was a major factor in weakening Roseto's characteristic family solidarity, the former unconditional support of family members certainly had weakened. When we studied Roseto in the early 1960s, although there were those who were in financial straights, no one was or had been on state or federal relief. Not until early 1980 did any Rosetan apply for social security disability benefits. Between 1984 and 1991 seven Rosetans did so, however, including two sons of the 92-year-old woman mentioned above and one of her daughters-in-law. Both boys had been in the group below age 35 during our first survey. When the seven were asked why they had not been helped by their families according to

Roseto's long tradition of keeping their people off welfare, there were two repeated responses: "I was too proud to ask my relatives for help," or "You don't understand, doctor; things have changed. People don't care."

9

Coda

Edward Gibbon, in his book, *The Decline and Fall of the Roman Empire*[117] wrote of a population whose citizens had become insensitive to their civil responsibilities, being more concerned about their livelihood than with contributing to their society. Referring to the Athenians he said, "In the end more than they wanted freedom, they wanted security, they wanted a comfortable life and in their quest for it all, security, comfort, freedom, they lost it all. When what the Athenians wanted finally was not to give to society but for society to give to them; when the freedom they wished for most was the freedom from responsibility, then Athenians ceased to be free."

There are elements of the Roseto story that, during the short interval of a hundred years, parallel in miniature the history of great powers in ancient Western civilization, Greece and Rome. In each case there was a coming together under early influence of inspirational leaders, followed by a period of comfortable prosperity. Ultimately, there developed signs of self-indulgence with a weakening of commitment to traditional values and a lack of responsibility for the community.

In the case of Roseto, the authors have tried not only to chronicle the relevant events, the forces behind them, and the collective and individual responses to them but also to illuminate to some extent the underlying social and neurobiological mechanisms at work. The evidence at hand confirms a familiar belief that whether a community lives in social equilibrium or social disruption depends on the way people treat each other as they cope with everyday challenges. It also strongly suggests that the way individuals perceive themselves and their role in society may palpably influence their health and that of their community.

Italian immigrants from Roseto Val Fortore and nearby towns arrived in Pennsylvania toward the end of the nineteenth century and settled on a hilltop, once a forest, that had been lumbered off to become an expanse of stumps and stones. It was the cheapest land available near the slate quarries, where the men worked ten- hour days to raise money enough to bring their wives and families to America. This was the physical scene that greeted Father de Nisco when, at the belated behest of Bishop Ryan, he arrived in 1896. The new community was, for the most part, in social turmoil, laced with crime, hooliganism, and fights that ended in stabbings. Father de Nisco's persistent exhortations, coupled with his personal generosity, encouragement, and practical assistance, shaped the community and its people into a close-knit, unostentatious but proud, and shortly to become incorporated town.

Roseto still bore the stamp of Father de Nisco when our study began in 1962, but it was less self-contained than it had been twenty years earlier. Fewer local businesses were able to survive as contacts with, and dependence on, the larger community of Eastern Pennsylvania increased. Rosetans were enjoying prosperity and respect instead of the former contempt from its neighbors. The protective need for community and family cohesion was less evident, and the years of suffering from social discrimination, exploitation, and poverty now seemed remote. Indications of changing values were evident in the new generation of young adults. Old social rules and taboos were weakening; values were changing among the new generation of young adults. Four years after our prediction that abandonment of Roseto's traditional attitudes and behavior would be accompanied by a rise in the death rate from heart attack, the first young Rosetan succumbed to a myocardial infarction. His story which appears in chapter 5, provides an extreme example of the changes in social perceptions that have occurred in Roseto. It also serves as a harbinger of the soon-to-be experienced rising death toll from coronary heart disease. The rapid and radical shifts in social standards and beliefs seem to have produced their effects with comparable swiftness.

New knowledge of the circuitry in the human brain may help explain in part how, in a genetically, ethnically, and socially homogeneous community, radical change can occur with such striking medical consequences. The mystery of what goes on in brain mechanisms when human beings are influenced by other human beings alone or in groups is being gradually unravelled. The impact of a sensation or an experience can be measured in lumens of light, decibels of sound, degrees of temperatures, and other physical units, but such refinements prove to be more or less irrelevant. The message itself, "What it means to me," although not quanitifiable, is what activates the structures in the brain that appraise the experience and formulate responses to it.

There is now clear evidence that afferent (incoming) impulses from sensory receptors of all sorts, on entering the brain, recruit a multitude of excitatory and inhibitory connections (dendritic synapses) from neurons that transmit information from circuits in thalamic, limbic, and cortical structures, where data from earlier learning experiences, biases, emotions, and beliefs are stored. Thus the original sensory message is shaped, intensified or moderated to elicit a strictly individual response in terms of emotion, understanding, and/or visceral and somatic behavior. Such central processing of information from afferent neurons generates individually specific conscious or unconscious perceptions that may, through autonomic effectors, direct and govern metabolic and thermodynamic functions, thereby altering the distribution of receptors, the synthesis of messenger molecules, and even gene expression in peripheral tissues. The steps involved in the formulation of a response to sensory signals from a personal encounter, either threatening or supportive, begin with the stimulation of sensory endings, visual, auditory, tactile, or otherwise. Thus sights, sounds, odors, tastes, touches, pains, pressures, and "vibes" from human relationships convey their messages, thereby discharging the "condensers" of the sensory nerves, which, in turn, transmit electrical energy via subsequent nerve connections into the brain and throughout manifold intercommunicating circuits that draw on stored memories, experiences, ingrained attitudes, values and standards, desires, aspirations, beliefs, algorithms of logic, and potentially everything previously learned.

There is a "receiving" area of the brain for most sensations: the olfactory bulb for olfactory messages the cochlear nucleus for sounds, the nucleus of the tractus solitarious for visceral afferent information, and so on. Having entered the substance of the brain, the afferent impulses encounter the influence of other neurons, either excitatory or inhibitory from elsewhere in a widespread neural circuit. The original message may be intensified, modulated, or even blocked as, for example, a sound may be "turned off" at the cochlear nucleus by inhibitory impulses from the cortex when an individual is engaging in mental concentration.[118] If the impulse survives the initial "way station" on entering the brain, it becomes subject to further modifying influences from stored or fresh information from elsewhere in the interactive circuitry between thalamus, reticular activating system, locus ceruleus, amygdala, limbic system, and various involved areas of the cortex. Within the same tiny fraction of time, the modified information is assessed, presumably in the frontal cortex. The behavioral decision that results from all this scanning and processing may include the activation of efferent pathways that act on the heart, vessels and other organs or on the tissues of the endocrine, immune, and other bodily systems.

Thus impressions from the environment, and especially from human relationships, immediate and remote, can powerfully shape many cognitive and behavioral aspects of a person. The salubrious social environment in Roseto created through the efforts of Father de Nisco certainly induced, among his fellow citizens, a perception of being emotionally sustained and nourished. In response, they seem to have sharpened their concern for one another and for the welfare of their community. As a result, individual responses to otherwise stressful life experiences may have been muted as the assessment of potentially troublesome events by evaluative circuits in their brain were influenced by their sense of confidence, self-esteem, purposefullness, and well-being. Years later, as necessity gave way to plenty and competition began to replace common purpose, new and more selfish influences were available to entrain the interpretive circuits of the brain and consequently the workings of the body.

The idea that one's perception of a life experience, or even one's state of mind, may participate in determining the health and behavior of bodily structures is not new; it was contained in the teachings of ancient philosophers. Later, the physician-philosopher, John Locke,[119] apparently influenced by the seventeenth century French philosopher Pierre Gassendi,[120] proposed a theory that all thought and behavior, somatic and visceral, are actuated by sensation (or experience), and that during the processing of sensations by the brain, the resulting behaviors are being shaped by stored attitudes, beliefs, biases, and learning, as well as the nature of an immediate experience itself. The theory was further supported when, in the early nineteenth century, Claude Bernard developed the view that a disease state reflected too much or too little adaptation to the environment on the part of the organ system of the body.[121]

Then in 1900 Charles Richet, professor of physiology in the Faculté de Médecine in Paris, proposed that "the protection of the organism" was achieved by regulatory mechanisms located in the brain. "The living being is stable," he wrote "It must be so in order not to be destroyed, dissolved or disintegrated by the colossal forces, often adverse, which surround it.... In a sense it is stable because it is modifiable—the slight instability is the necessary condition for the true stability of the organism." [122] In 1925 Cannon introduced his own concept of homeostasis with the above quote from Richet.[123] Ratcliffe, one-time director of the Penrose Research Laboratory at the Philadelphia Zoo, and Snyder reported a sharp increase in myocardial infarction among several species of birds and mammals independent of diet and age, but following a radical social change when new living arrangements were imposed by the staff on the 300 that were intended to control breeding pairs and groups.[124] In another study he found that his monkeys normally harbor pathogenic parasites but get sick from them only in the presence of an environmental stress such as being moved from one compound to another. Perhaps the human experience with the herpes simplex virus provides a comparable circumstance.[125]

Thus the potential for disease of Pasteur's microbes appears to depend, in part, on the effectiveness of bodily mechanisms, immunologic, endocrinologic, circulatory, and secretory, that protect the organism's mechanisms that are ultimately under the control of the brain.[126] To a great extent, therefore, the capability to be sick or well lies within us, in the capacity of our neuroregulatory mechanisms to respond appropriately.

Pasteur, upon his induction into the most lofty of French institutions, the Académie Française, declared that matters involving the emotions were not susceptible to scientific inquiry.[127] Although science still has not developed the means to study and understand the spiritual qualities of man, the scientist can nevertheless recognize and describe them, and now it is clear that the brain takes them into account in the process of evaluating experience and ordering all manner of responses, salutary and unsalutary.

There is ample evidence that the nourishment of the spirit is relevant to bodily health and performance. At Western Electric, when the company officials wanted to find out whether fluorescent lighting would increase the efficiency of working girls, they installed it in one of the workrooms. The productivity of the group working in that room soon exceeded the productivity of all other groups. Then it was suggested that the girls might do even better if the walls were painted a pastel shade. That also worked. Really interested by now, the management decided to test the effect of increasing the height of the workbenches by six inches. Again productivity increased, but then it was discovered that lowering the workbenches by six inches had the same effect. Ultimately it became clear to the officials that what was helping these workers toward better achievement was the recognition that someone was interested in their welfare and comfort.[128]

Another famous experiment was carried out by Frederick the Great in a foundling hospital in Germany. To cut down the mortality rate by eliminating germs, insofar as possible, he is said to have ordered the hospital attendants to change the babies' linen frequently, to keep things scrupulously clean, and to feed the children promptly but without holding or cuddling them in any way. Thus he hoped to avoid communicable diseases. Surprisingly, however, the lack of human warmth and loving resulted in the death of most of the babies, although at autopsy there were no specific lesions discernible. More recent observations among institutionalized infants have provided vivid confirmation of the hazards of lack of human warmth.[129]

How often have we seen the broken spirit of the elderly lead to their deterioration and death when they no longer felt wanted or useful. Dr. Calvin Plimpton, the president of Amherst College, tells the story of a man who died and shortly thereafter found himself transported to a delightfully cool and comfortable spot where his every want was supplied as soon as he mentioned it. In fact, one of the angels, who appeared to be assigned to him, continually asked him what he would like to have in order to raise his level of enjoyment. He asked for, and received, a fine house with a kidney-shaped swimming pool, a sports car, and a few lovely young ladies in addition to a wealth of luxury items. At this point he was having difficulty deciding what else he wanted. One day he asked, "Isn't there some work I could do around here?" The angel replied, "Oh, gracious, no! There's no work." "Well, couldn't I be useful in some way? Isn't there something I could help out with?" There seemed to be no opportunities along this line at all. Becoming more and more restless, the man kept imploring the angel for some little thing he might undertake in the way of work, but always with the same reply. Finally in exasperation he said, "Well, if it's going to go on like this indefinitely, I would have preferred to go to Hell." "And just where," said the angel, "do you think you are?"

The study of the lofty aspects of man's spirit should prove as interesting and as fruitful as the study of his more earthy qualities. It might, in fact, be the new frontier for medicine.

Appendix
Results of the Structured Interview
Used in the 1966 Visits to 86 Percent of
the Homes in Roseto

At the time of the visit, 904 individuals, 431 men and 473 women between the ages of 18 and 99 were interviewed at home. The topics covered (attached form) were approximately identical to those in the sociological interviews conducted as part of the 1962-63 individual survey in which many of those who were visited had participated. Statements made in these interviews already gave evidence of change in social attitudes and values. Since we had predicted the likelihood of an increase in prevalence of and mortality from, myocardial infarction in Roseto, each subject was followed for 25 years to outcome in 1991.

One hundred nineteen, 78 men and 41 women among those interviewed experienced a myocardial infarction at some time during the succeeding 25 years. Of that group 19 men and 9 women survived the infarction but for 59 of the men and 32 of the women the infarction had proved fatal (see table A-1). The mean age of the survivors was 49 and that of the decendents 58.

To ascertain whether or not answers to questions made in the interviews might have suggested the likelihood of a subsequent infarct, all 119 subjects who later experienced myocardial infarction were individually matched for age and sex with controls who had remained healthy. The statistical significance of differences was calculated by the chi square method on 44 selected variables contained in the 130 covered in the interview.

While a great deal of useful information was garnered from the statements made by the subjects during the interviews, in only 3 of the categories that had been selected for comparison,—education, family and general (personal)—did the replies to specific questions differentiate at a statistically significant level of confidence those destined to experience myocardial infarction over the next 25 years from their matched controls who remained healthy throughout. All 3 significant questions had to do with personal commitments and responsibilities as follows:

Question No. 15, "Subject's last grade completed in school." Those individuals who later experienced myocardial infarction had had more formal education than their matched controls. p = .05.

Question No. 70, "Who would you say is the person your family depends on most (the person who solves most of the family problems). Those destined to die of myocardial infarction felt that they themselves were the person most depended on by family members, while matched controls mentioned others. p = 0.05.

Question No. 97, "What things could cause you to worry?"

Those who later suffered fatal myocardial infarction worried mainly about their own children and other living family members, while their controls were more inclined to worry about illness or death of a relative. p = .02.

Table A-1
Analysis of Groups Matched by Sex and Age

Myocardial Infarction	Matched Controls	Totals
Survived		
N = 28	N = 28	N = 56
M 19 F9	M 19 F 9	M 38 F 18
Died		
N = 91	N = 91	N = 182
M 59 F 32	M 59 F 32	M 188 F 64
Totals		
N = 119	N = 119	N = 238
M 78 F 41	M 78 F 41	M 156 F 82

Sociological Data
Roseto, Pennsylvania
(Summer, 1966)

Interviewer's Name
_____

_____Code No.
1-4

_____Date of Interview _____
5-10   Day,   Month,   Year

         Subject's Name _____

         Subject's Address _____
                          House No.   Street   Town

                          ****

_____1. Sex   M   F
11

_____2. Marital Status   a) single   b) married   c) remarried
12
                              d) divorced   d) separated   f) widowed

_____3. Age at first marriage   Inapplicable (if single) _____
13-14

_____4. Number of children   Inapplicable (if single) _____
15

                              AGE

_____5. Subject's Age _____
16-17

_____6. Subject's Age Group _____ (leave blank)
18

_____7. Spouse's Age _____
19-20

                    ETHNIC IDENTIFICATION

_____8. Subject's Ethnic Identification   Italian _____
21   Other (specify) _____

_____9. Spouse's Ethnic Identification   Italian _____
22   Other (specify) _____

BIRTHPLACE

_____ 10. Subject's Birthplace a) Roseto, PA b) Roseto, Italy c) Other (specify)
23   _____

_____ 11. Spouse's Birthplace   a) Roseto, PA b) Roseto, Italy c) Other (specify)
24   _____

_____ 12. Subject's Father's Birthplace a) Roseto, PA b) Roseto, Italy
25   c) Other (specify) _____

RELIGION

_____ 13. Subject's Religion a)Roman Catholic b)Presbyterian c)Jeh. Witness
26
                               d)Other (specify) _____ e) None

_____ 14. Spouse's Religion a)Roman Catholic b)Presbyterian c)Jeh. Witness
27
                               d) Other (specify) _____ e) None

EDUCATION

_____ 15. Subject's Education _____
28-29   Last grade completed in school

_____ 16. Spouse's Education _____
30-31   Last grade completed in school

        17. Subject's Father's Education _____
                                         Last grade completed in school

OCCUPATION

_____ 18. Subject's Present Occupation _____
32
            If unemployed or retired, usual occupation _____

            Description of present or usual occupation _____

            _____
                    Duties, skills required, etc.

_____ 19. Spouse's Present Occupation _____
33
            If unemployed or retired, usual occupation _____

            Description of present or usual occupation _____

            _____
                    Duties, skills requried, etc.

        20. Subject's Father's Present or Usual Occupation _____

_____ 21. Subject's Social Class _____ (leave blank)
34

_____ 22. Subject's Educational Mobility _____ (leave blank)
35-37

_____ 23. Subject's Occupational Mobility _____ (leave blank)
38-40

WORK HISTORY AND JOB CONTINUITY

_____ 24. Subject's Work History (list all major full-time jobs during last
41   20 years) (Start with present job and work backwards)

	Type of Job	Length of Time Held	Why Changed Jobs
1.			
2.			
3.			
4.			
5.			
6.			
7.			
8.			
9.			
10.			

_____ 25. Spouse's Work History (list all major full-time jobs during last
42   20 years) (Start with present job and work backwards)

1.			
2.			
3.			
4.			
5.			
6.			
7.			
8.			
9.			
10.			

TWO JOBS OR OVERTIME

_____ 26. Subject presently working on two jobs?   Yes   No
43

_____ 27. How many hours a week do you work in your job?_____ hrs/wk
44

_____ 28. If overtime, is this because he has to or own choice?_____
45

_____ 29. Do you work in Roseto, Bangor or in another town? _____
46   (specify town)

_____ 30. Spouse presently working at two jobs?   Yes   No
47

_____ 31. How many hours a week does your spouse work in his job? _____hrs/wk
48

_____ 32. If overtime, is this because he has to or own choice? _____
49

_____ 33. Does your spouse work in Roseto, Bangor or another town? _____
50   (specify towr

RESIDENTIAL HISTORY

_____ 34. How long has subject lived in Roseto, PA? _____
51

Where did subject live before he moved to Roseto, PA _____
                                                      town & state
How long did he live there? _____

Was there any special reason why you moved to Roseto? _____

_____ 35. How long has spouse lived in Roseto, PA?_____
52

Where did spouse live before he moved to Roseto, PA _____
                                                     town & state
How long did he live there?

PRESENT LIVING ARRANGEMENTS

_____ 36. Who lives with you in your present house (or apartment)?
53

_____

_____

INCOME

_____ 37. Subject's present gross yearly income $ _____
54-58

_____ 38. Spouse's present gross yearly income $_____
59-63

_____ 39. Subject and Spouse present combined income $_____
64-68

_____ 40. Peak income (most subject ever earned in one year) _____ Year____
69-73

LEISURE TIME

_____ 41. What is your favorite way of spending your leisure (free) time?
74
_____

_____

_____ 42. What is your spouse's favorite way of spending his leisure (free) time
75
_____

_____

_____ 43. How many nights a week, on average, do you spend away from home?
76
(for example, at the clubs) _____

_____ 44. How many nights a week, on average, does your spouse spend away
77
from home? _____

_____ 45. In your opinion, how do most of the men in Roseto spend their
78
leisure time? _____

_____

_____ 46. In your opinion, how do most of the women in Roseto spend their
79
leisure time? _____

_____

_____ Card No. 1
80
Begin Card No. 2 (Reproduce columns 1-40)

SMOKING

_____ 47. Does subject smoke now?　　　　　　Yes　　　No
41

　　　　If _yes_, what and how much?　Cigarettes _____
　　　　　　　　　　　　　　　　　　　　　　　　　　　quantity
　　　　　　　　　　　　　　　　　　Cigars　　_____
　　　　　　　　　　　　　　　　　　　　　　　　　　　quantity
　　　　　　　　　　　　　　　　　　Pipe　　　_____
　　　　　　　　　　　　　　　　　　　　　　　　　　　quantity

　　　　How many years have you smoked? _____

_____ 48. When do you smoke the most? (at work, home, socially, etc) _____
42

_____ 49. If _no_, have you ever smoked?　　　Yes　　　No
43

　　　　Why quit? _____

_____ 50. Does spouse smoke now?　　　Yes　　　No
44

　　　　If _yes,_ what and how much?　Cigarettes _____
　　　　　　　　　　　　　　　　　　　　　　　　　　　quantity
　　　　　　　　　　　　　　　　　　Cigars　　_____
　　　　　　　　　　　　　　　　　　　　　　　　　　　quantity
　　　　　　　　　　　　　　　　　　Pipe　　　_____
　　　　　　　　　　　　　　　　　　　　　　　　　　　quantity
　　　　How many years has your spouse smoked? _____

_____ 51. When does your spouse smoke the most? (at work, home, socially, etc)
45

　　　　_____

_____ 52. If _no_, has your spouse ever smoked?　　　Yes　　　No
46

　　　　Why quit? _____

ORGANIZATIONAL MEMBERSHIP

_____ 53. Are you a member of any clubs, lodges, unions, political, religious
47 　　　or civic organizations now?　　　Yes　　　No

_____ 54. In which of the above is he most active? _____
48 　　　　　　　　　　　　　　　　　　　　　Name of organization

_____ 55. Has subject held any offices in any of these organizations? Yes　No
49

_____ 56. Is spouse a member of any clubs, lodges, unions, political, religious
50 　　　or civic organizations now?　　　Yes　　　No

_____ 57. In which of the above is spouse _most_ active? _____
51 　　　　　　　　　　　　　　　　　　　　　Name of organization

_____58. Has spouse held any offies in any of these organizations? Yes NO
52

_____59. In your opinion, what do you consider the most important organization
53   to belong to in Roseto? _____
                                  Name of organization
          In what ways do you think this organization is important? _____

          _____

_____60. Do you think it is necessary to be active in organizations in
54   Roseto?   Yes   No

                    CHILDREN (omit if subject is single)
_____61. How many of your children are living at home now? _____
55

_____62. How many of your children have moved away from Roseto? _____
56

_____63. Have any of your children graduated from college?   Yes   No
57

_____64. Have any of your children married someone who is not an Italian?
58   Yes   No

_____65. In what ways do you think the children in Roseto today are different
59   from Roseto children, say 20 years ago?

          _____

          _____

          _____

_____66. Where do (or did) your child (or most of your children) go to grade
60   and high school?

                              _____Columbus Grade School

                              _____Pius High School

                              _____Bangor High School

                              _____Elsewhere (specify) _____

_____67. Who disciplines (punishes) your children? _____
61

          _____

FAMILY

_____68. If you had a problem, who is the person who you would want to talk
62   to about it? _____

_____69. Would you say that your closest friend lives in Roseto, Bangor or
63   elsewhere? _____

_____70. Who would you say is the person that your family depends upon the
64   most (the person who solves most of the family problems)?
            _____

_____71. Lets say, for example, that you were unhappy in your job. What
65   would you do? _____

            _____

            _____

            _____

_____72. In your opinion, what do you think most people do in Roseto when
66   they have family problems (troubles)?

            _____

            _____

            _____

_____73. Think now about the most unhappy or upsetting time in your life.
67   (Probe to get nature of situation. Describe below).

            _____

            _____

            _____

            What did you do to help you handle this problem?

            _____

            _____

            _____

            _____

_____ 74. Did your religion help you in any way in handling this problem?
68
_____

_____

_____

_____ 75. What would you say is one of the most unhappy or upsetting things
69   that could happen to you or your family?

_____

_____

_____

COMMUNITY--POWER STRUCTURE

_____ 76. Who do you think is the most influential person in Roseto today?
70
_____

_____ 77. What clan or family do you feel is the most influential in
71   in Roseto today? _____

_____ 78. What do you think are the main things that make a person or family
72   important or influential in Roseto today? (For example, money,
        political affiliation, knowing the right people, means used in
        getting ahead, education, religious affiliation, etc.)

_____

_____

_____

_____

_____ 79. Do you think there are some persons living in Roseto that don't
73   "fit in" with the rest of the town?   Yes   No

        If yes, in what way don't they "fit in?" _____

_____

_____

_____

HANDLING PROBLEMS

_____80. Is it easy or difficult for you to relax?   Easy   Difficult
74
If easy, what do you do to relax? _____

_____

If difficult, why do you think you have difficulty relaxing?

_____

_____

_____

_____

_____81. Would you say that you are usually tense?   Yes   No
75
If yes, is there any particular reason? _____

_____

_____82. Do you get physical exercise every day?   Yes   No
76
If yes, what kind of exercise? _____

_____

_____83. Would you say that you are usually nervous?   Yes   No
77
If yes, is there any particular reason why you think you

are nervous? _____

_____84. Have you been able to do what you wanted to do in life? Yes   No
78
Comments: _____

_____

_____85. Do you eat foods that are different from those that your parents
79
ate?   Yes   No

If yes, how have your eating patterns changed? (Particular foods,
method of preparation, etc.)

_____

_____

_____

_____

<u>2</u>　　Card No. 2
<u>80</u>

Begin Card No. 3 (Reproduce Columns 1-40)

_____86. Do you eat: a) only Italian foods; b) some Italian, some American;
<u>41</u>　　　c) only American foods? _____

_____87. Do you make your own wine?　Yes　　No
<u>42</u>

_____88. How many glasses of wine do you have every day or week?
<u>43</u>　　　　　　　　　　　_____ None

　　　　　　　　　　　_____ Glasses per day

　　　　　　　　　　　_____ Glasses per week

_____89. Do you drink beer or liquor?　____Beer____Liquor____Both____None
<u>44</u>　　　If yes, how often and how much? _____
　　　　　　　　　　　　　　　　(frequency and amount)

_____90. Do you eat more when you are worried, tense or nervous? Yes　　No
<u>45</u>

_____91. Do you eat less when you are depressed or tired?　Yes　　No
<u>46</u>

_____92. Have you changed your way of eating since our research team
<u>47</u>　　　came to Roseto in 1962?　Yes　　No

　　　If yes, in what ways? _____

　　　_____

ILLNESSES

_____93. Have you had (or do you now have) any of the following:
<u>48</u>

　　　Frequent headaches _____　　Ulcers _____　High Blood Pressure _____

　　　Heart Attack _____　Frequent chest pains _____　Others _____

_____94. Have you taken (or now take) pills to help you sleep? Yes　　No
<u>49</u>

_____95. Have you taken (or now take) pills for your nerves? Yes　　No
<u>50</u>

GENERAL QUESTIONS

_____96. Have you ever thought about moving away from Roseto?　Yes　　No
<u>51</u>　　　If yes, Why? _____

　　　_____

_____97. What things could cause you to worry? _____
  52   _____
          _____

_____98. Do you ever leave Roseto? _____
  53   For what reasons? _____
          _____

_____99. Do you think people who have moved away from Roseto are different
  54   in any way from those people who have stayed in Roseto? Yes   No
          If yes, in what ways are they different? _____
          _____
          _____

_____100. When is the last time you went to see a doctor? _____
  55   (month & year)
           Reason: _____

_____101. Do you have any brothers or sisters? _____
  56   (No. brothers) (No. Sisters)

_____102. If yes, how many live in Roseto? _____
  57   (No. brothers) (No. Sisters)

_____103. Regarding those living elsewhere:
  58   Where Live   Type of Work   Did they ever live in Roseto
                                                      Yes   No
           1. _____ _____ _____
           2. _____ _____ _____
           3. _____ _____ _____
           4. _____ _____ _____
           5. _____ _____ _____

_____104. How do you think most people in Roseto feel about someone in Roseto
  59   being divorced?
          _____
          _____

_____105. How do you think most people in Roseto feel about someone who
  60   marries a person who is not an Italian?
          _____
          _____
          _____

_____106. Do you think most Rosetans want to keep Roseto a town for
61   Italians   Yes   No

Comments: _____

_____

_____

_____107. Did you come to any of the Oklahoma University Medical Clinics?
62   Yes   No

If no, are there any reasons why you didn't come? _____

_____

_____108. Does your clan have reunions?   Yes   No
63

If yes, did you go to the last reunion?   Yes   No

Which clan in Roseto has the most reunions? _____

_____109. If you had your choice of jobs would you choose a different job
64   from the one you have now?   Yes   No

_____110. What would you like to do (in life) that you are doing now?
65

_____

_____

_____

_____

References

1. Sadat, A. 1978. *In Search of Identity: An Autobiography*. New York: Harper and Row.
2. Donnison, C. P. 1938. *Civilization and Disease*. Baltimore: William Wood.
3. Brown, W. L. 1938. Introduction to *Civilization and Disease* by C. P. Donnison. Baltimore: William Wood.
4. Halliday, J. L. 1948. *Psychosocial Medicine: A Study of the Sick Society*. New York. W. W. Norton.
5. Simmons, L. W. and Wolff, H. G. 1954. Social Science in Medicine. New York: Russell Sage Foundation.
6. Dubos, R. 1951. Biological and social aspects of tuberculosis. *Bulletin of the New York Academy of Medicine*, 27:351.
7. Kannel, W. B. and Gordon, T. 1974. The Framingham Study. An epidemiological investigation of cardiovascular disease. Publication No. (NIH) 74-599. Washington, DC: Department of Health, Education and Welfare.
8. Friedman, M. and Rosenman, R. 1959. Association of specific overt behavior pattern with blood and cardiovascular findings. *JAMA*, 169:1286.
9. Kobhasa, S. C. 1990. Stress-resistant personality. In *The Healing Brain*, ed. Robert Ornstein and C. Swencionis. New York: Guilford Press.
10. Antonovsky, A. 1979. *Health, Stress, and Coping: New Perspectives on Mental and Physical Well-being*. San Francisco. Jossey-Bass.
11. Holmes, T. H. and Rahe, R. H. 1967. The social readjustment rating scale. *Journal Psychosomatic Research*, 11:213-218.
12. Lynch, J. J. 1979. *The Broken Heart: The Medical Consequences of Loneliness*. New York: Basic Books.
13. Karasek, R. A., Theorell, T., and Schwartz, P. J. 1982. Job, psychological factors and coronary heart disease. *Advances in Cardiology*, 29:62-67.
14. Kaplan, G. A., Salonen, J. T., Cohe, R. D., Brand, R. J., Syme, S. L., and Puska, P. 1988. Social connections and mortality from all causes and from cardiovascular disease: Prospective evidence from eastern Finland. *American Journal of Epidemiology*, 128(2):370-380.
15. Berkman, L., and Syme, S. 1979. Social networks, host resistance and mortality. A nine-year follow-up study of Alameda County residents. *American Journal of Epidemiology*, 109:186-204.
16. Cassel, J. 1976. The contribution of the social environment to host resistance. *American Journal of Epidemiology*, 104:107-113.
17. Brunner, D., Meshulam, N., Altman, S., Bearman, J.E., Lobbl, K., and Wendkos, M. E. 1971. Physiologic and anthropometric parameters related to coronary risk factors in Yemenite Jews living different time spans in Israel. *Journal Chronic Diseases*, 24:383-392. Also, personal communication.
18. Uehlinger, E. 1970. Den krankheitswert der beginnenden. In S. Likos, ed. *Internationl Archiv fur Arbeitsmedizin*, 26:1-30.
19. Seguin, C. A. 1956. Migration and psychosomatic disadaptation. *Journal of Psychosomatic Medicine*, 18:404.

20. Wolf, S. and Wolf, T. 1978. A preliminary study in medical anthropology in Brunei, Borneo. *Pavlovian Journal of Biological Science*, 13:42-54.
21. Bruhn, J. G., and Wolf, S. 1978. *The Roseto Story: An Anatomy of Health*, Norman: University of Oklahoma Press.
22. Romano, D. 1965. *I've Got to Work Till I Die*. New York: Vantage Press.
23. Barzini, L. 1964. *The Italians*. New York: Atheneum, p. 292.
24. *Encyclopaedia Britannica*. 1911. 11th ed., vol. 14:27-44, New York: Cambridge University Press.
25. Facchiano, A. 1971. *Roseto Val Fortore*. Brussels: Indagini Storiche.
26. Goethe, W. 1962. *Italian Journey 1786-1788*. Introduction by W. H. Auden and translated by Elizabeth Mayer. New York: Pantheon Books.
27. Wolf, S., Grace, K. L., Bruhn, J. G., and Stout, C. 1973. Roseto revisited: Further data on the incidence of myocardial infarction in Roseto and neighboring Pennsylvania communities. *Transactions of the American Clinical and Climatological Association*, 85:100-108.
28. Carter, M. H. 1908. One man and his town. *McClure's Magazine*, 30:275-286.
29. *San Francisco Chronicle*, June 5, 1964. The town that really lives (unsigned).
30. Oppedisano, R. 1977. Roseto revisited. *The National Magazine for Italian Americans*. February, p. 38.
31. Basso, R. 1952. *History of Roseto*. Easton, PA: Tanzella Printing.
32. Valletta, C. L. 1973. *The Settlement of Roseto: World View and Promise*. In *The Ethnic Experience in Pennsylvania*, ed. J. E. Bodnar, Lewisburg, PA: Bucknell University Press, p. 123.
33. Valletta, C. L. 1975 *A Study of Americanization in Carneta*. New York: Arno Press.
34. Bianca, C. 1974. *The Two Rosetos*. Bloomington: Indiana University Press.
35. Lord, T.J.D., and Barrows, S. J. 1906. *The Italian in America*, New York: B. F. Buck.
36. Bruhn, J. G., Philips, B. U., and Wolf, S. 1972. Social readjustment and illness patterns: Comparisons between first, second, and third generation Italian-Americans living in the same community. *Journal Psychosomatic Research*, 16:387-394.
37. Gans, H. J. 1962. *The Urban Villagers*. IL: Free Press.
38. Wolf, S. and Goodell, H. 1968. *Stress and Disease*, 2nd ed. Springfield, IL: Charles C. Thomas.
39. Pocock, S. J., Shaper, A. G., Cook, D. G., Phillips, A. N., and Walter, M. 1987. Social class differences in ischemic heart disease in British men. *Lancet*, ii:197-201.
40. Williams, R. 1989. *The Trusting Heart: Great News About Type A Behavior*. New York: Random House
41. Cohen, S., and Syme, L. S. 1985. Issues in the study and application of support, In Cohen, S. C. and Syme, L. S. (eds.) *Social Support and Health*, pp. 3-72, New York: Academic Press.
42. Groen, J. J. 1977. Psychosomatic aspects of ischemic (coronary) heart disease. In *Modern Trends: Psychosomatic Medicine*, O. Hill (ed.), vol. 3, London: Butterworth, Barton and Lawn, pp. 289-329.
43. Von Dusch, T. 1868. *Lehrbuch der Herzkronkheiten Leipzig*. Verlag Von Wilhelm Engelman.
44. Osler, W. 1910. The Lumelian Lectures on angina pectoris. *Lancet*, 1:839-844.
45. Stout, C., Morrow, J., Brandt, E. N. and Wolf, S. 1964. Study of an Italian community in Pennsylvania. Unusually low incidence of death from myocardial infarction. *JAMA*, 188:845-849.

46. Brandt, E. N., Stout, C., Hampton, J. W., Lynn, T. N. and Wolf, S. 1966. Coronary heart disease among Italians and non-Italians in Roseto, Pennsylvania, and nearby communities. In: *Prevention of Ischemic Heart Disease: Principles and Practices*, Rabb, W., ed., pp. 1-9, Springfield, IL: Charles C. Thomas.
47. Kiritz, S. and Moss, R. H. 1974. Physiological effects of social circumstances. *Psychosomatic Medicine*, 3:96-114.
48. Spittle, B. and James, B. 1977. Psychosocial factors and myocardial infarction. *Australian/New Zealand Journal of Psychology*, 37:96-114.
49. Jenkins, C. D. 1978. Behavioral risk factors in coronary artery disease. *Heart Disease and Behavior*, 29:543-562.
50. Rahe, R. H. and Arthur, R. J. 1978. Life change and illness studies: Past history and future directions. *Journal of Human Stress*, 4:3-15.
51. Thoreson, R. W. and Ackerman, M. 1981. Research review: Cardiac rehabilitation: basic principles and psychosocial factors. *Rehabilitation Counsel Bulletin*, 24:223-255.
52. Schwab, J. J. 1986. Stress from a psychiatric epidemiological perspective. *Stress Medicine*, 2:211-220.
53. Keys, A. 1966. Arteriosclerotic heart disease in a favored community. *Journal of Chronic Diseases*, 19:245-254
54. Keys, A. 1966. Arteriosclerotic heart disease in Roseto, Pennsylvania. *JAMA*, 195:93-95.
55. Horan, P. M. and Gray, B. H. Status inconsistency, mobility and coronary heart disease. *Journal of Health and Social Behavior*, 151:300-310.
56. Wolf, S. 1966. Mortality from myocardial infarction in Roseto. *JAMA*, 2:195.
57. Egolf, B., Lasker, J., Wolf, S., and Potvin, L. The Roseto Effect: A 60-year comparison of mortality rates. *American Journal of Public Health*, in press 1992.
58. Wolf, S., Herrenkohl, R. C., Lasker, J., Egolf, G., Philips, B. U. and Bruhn, J. G. 1988. Roseto, Pennsylvania, 25 years later-highlights of a medical and sociological survey. *Transactions of the American Clinical and Climatological Association*, 100:57-67.
59. Thomas, C. B. 1976. Precursors of premature disease and death: The predictive potential of habits and family attitudes. *Annals of Internal Medicine*, 85:653-658.
60. Thomas, C. B. and Ross, D. C. 1968. Precursors of hypertension and coronary disease among healthy medical students. Discriminant function analysis V. Family Attitudes. *Johns Hopkins Medical Journal*, 123:283-296.
61. Thomas, C. B., and Duszynoki, K. R. 1974. Closeness to parents and the family constellation in a prospective study of 5 disease states: Suicide, mental illness, malignant tumors, hypertension, and coronary heart disease. *Johns Hopkins Medical Journal*, 134:251-270.
62. Kaplan, B. H., Cassel, J. C., and Gore, S. 1977. Social support and health. *Medical Care*, 15(5):47-59.
63. Gore, S. 1978. The effect of social support in moderating the health consequences of unemployment. *Journal of Health and Social Behavior*, 19:157-165.
64. Fuchs, V. 1975. *Who Shall Live?* New York: Basic Books.
65. Matsumoto, Y. S. 1970. Social stress and coronary heart disease in Japan: A hypothesis. *The Milbank Memorial Fund Quarterly.* 48:9-36.
66. Page, L. B., Damon, A., and Moellering, R. . 1974. Antecedents of cardiovascular disease in six Solomon Island societies. *Circulation*, 49:1132-1146.

67. Cassel, J., Patrick, R., and Jenkins, C. 1960. Epidemiological analysis of the health implications of culture change: A conceptual model. *Annals of the New York Academy of Sciences*, 84:938.

68. Obeyesekere, I. 1968. Evaluation of risk factors in coronary heart disease in Ceylon. Paper presented at the Fourth Asian Pacific Congress of Cardiology, Jerusalem and Tel Aviv, September 1-7.

69. Groover, M. E., Boone, L., Houk, P. and Wolf, S. 1967. Problems in the quantitation of dietary survey. *JAMA*, 201(1):8-10.

70. Boone, L. 1967. A study of the relationships between oral behavior, emotional stress and life events in patients with coronary heart disease. Master's thesis. University of Oklahoma.

71. Harris, S. S., Casperson, C. J., DeFriese, G. H., and Estes, E. H. Jr. 1989. Physical activity counseling for healthy adults as a primary prevention intervention in the clinical setting. Report for the U.S. Preventive Services Task Force. *JAMA*, 261:3588-3598.

72. Gordon, N. F., Scott, C. B. 1991. The role of exercise in the primary and secondary prevention of coronary heart disease. *Clinical Sports Medicine*, 10(1):87-103.

73. Perkanen, J., Linn, S., Heiss, G., Suchindran, C.M., Leon, A., Rifkind, B. M. and Tyroler, H. A. 1990. Ten-year mortality from cardiovascular disease in relation to cholesterol level among men with and without preexisting cardiovascular disease. *New England Journal of Medicine*, 322:1700-1707.

74. Imai, H., Taylor, C. B., and Werthessen, N. T. 1976. Angiotoxicity and arteriosclerosis due to contaminants of USP grade cholesterol. *Archives of Pathology and Laboratory Medicine*, 100:565-572.

75. Imai, H. 1977. Report of Workshop on Study and Review of Angiotoxic and Carcinogenic Sterols in Processed Food. Washington, DC: Army Research Office and Office of Naval Research.

76. Palinski, W., Rosenfeld, M. E., Yiä-Herttuala. 1989. Low-density lipoprotein undergoes oxidative modification in vivo. *Proceedings of the National Academy of Sciences of the United States of America*, 86:1372-1376.

77. Mitchinson, M. J., Ball, R. Y., Carpenter, K. L. H., and Parums, D. V. 1988. Macrophages and ceroid in atherosclerosis. In K.E. Suckling and P. H. E. Groot, eds., *Hyperlipadaemia and Atherosclerosis*, London: Academic Press, pp. 117-134.

78. Smith, L. L., Mathews, W. S., and Price, J. C. 1967. Thin layer chromatographic examination of cholesterol autoxidation. *Journal of Chromatography*, 187-205.

79. Peng, S. K., and Taylor, C. B. Cholesterol Autoxidation. In *Rural Review of Nutrition and Dietetics*, ed. Bourne, E., vol. 44 117-154. Basel: Karger.

80. Mann, G. 1974. Hypothesis: The role of vitamin C in diabetic angiopathy. *Perspectives in Biology and Medicine*, Winter, 210-216.

81. Verlangier, A. J. and Sestito, J. 1981. Effect of insulin on ascorbic acid uptake by heart endothelial cells: Possible relationship to retinal atherogenesis. *Life Sciences*, 29:5-9.

82. Pikul, J., and Kummerow, F. A. 1990. Lipid oxidation in chicken muscles and skin after roasting and refrigerated storage and main broiler parts. *Journal of Food Sciences*, 55(1)30-37.

83. Liu, J., Simon, L. M., Philips, J. R. and Robin, E. D. 1977. Superoxide dismutase activity in hypoxic mammalian systems. *Journal of Applied Physiology*, 42:107-110.

84. Kandutsch, A. A., Heiniger, J.J., and Chen, H. W. 1977. Effects of 25-hydroxycholesterol and 7-ketocholesterol inhibitors of sterol synthesis, administered orally to mice. *Biochim, biophys. Acta*, 486:260-272.

85. Lynn, T., Duncan, R., Naughton, J. P., Brandt, E., Wulff, J., Wolf, S., McCabe, W. R., Yamamoto, J., Adsett, C. A. and Schottstaedt, W. W. 1962. Changes in serum lipids in relation to emotional stress during rigid control of diet and exercise. *Transactions of the American Clinical and Climatological Association*. 73:162. Also, *Circulation*, 26(3): 379.

86. Groen, J. J., Tijong, B. K. and Willebrands, A. F. 1952. Influence of nutrition, individuality and various forms of stress on serum cholesterol: Results of an experiment of 9 months duration in 60 normal volunteers. *Netherlands Journal of Nutrition*, 13:556-572.

87. Thomas, C. B., and Murphy, E. A. 1958. Further studies on cholesterol levels in the Johns Hopkins medical students: Effect of stress at examinations. *Journal of Chronic Diseases*, 8:661.

88. Wertlake, P. T., Wilcox, A. A., Haley, M. I., Peterson, J. E. 1958. Relationship of mental and emotional stress to serum cholesterol levels. *Proceedings of the Society of Experimental Biology and Medicine*, 97:163.

89. Grundy, S. N., Griffin, A. C., 1959. Effects of periodic mental stress on serum cholesterol levels. *Circulation*, 19:496.

90. Dreyfuss, F., and Czackes, J.W. 1959. Blood cholesterol and uric acid of healthy medical students under stress of an examination. *Archives of Internal Medicine*, 103:708.

91. Rahe, R. H., Rubin, R. T., Arther, R. J., and Clark, B. R. 1968. Serum uric acid and cholesterol variability: A comprehensive view of underwater demolition team training. *JAMA* 206:2875-2880.

92. Groover, M. E., Jr. 1957. Clinical evaluation of a public health program to prevent coronary artery disease. *Transactions of the College of Physicians*, 24:105.

93. Friedman, M., Rosenmann, R. H. and Carroll, V. 1958. Changes in the serum cholesterol and blood clotting time in men subjected to cyclic variation of occupational stress. *Circulation* 17:852.

94. Hammersten, J. F., Cathey, C., Redmond, R. F. and Wolf, S. 1957. Serum cholesterol, diet and stress in patients with coronary artery disease. *Journal of Clinical Investigation* (Abstract), 36:897.

95. Wolf, S. 1976. Sinus Arrhythmia: A Biologic Rhythm with Complex Determinants. In honor of Thomas Doxiadis, pp. 609-614, Athens, Greece.

96. Wenkebach, K. F., and Winterberg, I. I. 1927. *Die unregelmassige Herztatigkeit*. Leipzig: Engelman.

97. Sherf, D., and Boyd, L. J. 1946. *Clinical Electrocardiography*. Philadelphia: Lippincott.

98. Gross, D. 1962. The clinical significance of sinus arrhythmia and angina pectoris. *Cardiologia*, 41:246-255.

99. Wolf, S. (ed.). 1971. *The Artery and the Process of Arteriosclerosis: Measurement and Modification*, S. Wolf ed. pp. 235-237, New York: Plenum Press.

100. Martin, C. J., Magid, N. M., Myers, G., Barnett, P., Schaad, J. W., Weiss, J. S., Lesch, M., and Singer, D. H. 1987. Heart rate variability and sudden death secondary to coronary artery disease during ambulatory electrocardiographic monitoring. *American Journal of Cardiology*, 60:86-89.

101. Cripps, T. R., Malik, M., Farrell, T. G. and Camm, A. J. 1991. Prognostic value of reduced heart rate variability after myocardial infarction: Clinical evaluation of a new analysis method. *British Heart Journal*, 65:14–19.
102. Schneider, R. A. and Costiloe, J. P. 1972. In: *The Artery and the Process of Arteriosclerosis*, ed. Wolf, S. New York: Plenum Press, p. 307.
103. Hampton, J. W., Mantooth, J., Brandt, E. N., and Wolf, S. 1966. Plasma fibrinogen patterns in patients with coronary atherosclerosis. *Circulation*, 34:1098–1101.
104. Stone, M. C. and Thorp, J. M. 1985. Plasma fibrinogen—a major coronary risk factor. *Journal of the Royal College General Practitioners*, 35:565–569.
105. Schwartz, P. and Wolf, S. 1978. QT interval prolongation as predictor of sudden death in patients with myocardial infarction. *Circulation*, 57(6):1074–1077.
106. Huang, M. H., Ebey, J. and Wolf, S. 1989. Responses of the QT interval of the electrocardiogram during emotional stress. *Psychosomatic Medicine*, 51:419–427.
107. Huang, M. H., Hull, S. S., Foreman, R. D., Lazzara, R., and Wolf, S. 1992. Heart rate-QT relationships during baroreceptor stimulation with diminished autonomic influence on ventricles. *Integrative Physiological and Behavioral Science*, Vol. 27.
108. Theorell, T., and Blunk, D. 1975. Ballistocardiographic measurements of the heart's force of contraction during two years preceding death from ischemic heart disease. *Journal of Laboratory and Clinical Medicine*, 86:46–56.
109. Wolf, S. and Goodell, H. 1976. *Behavioral Science in Clinical Medicine*, Springfield, IL, Charles C. Thomas, pp. 58–60.
110. Sevelius, G. (ed.). 1965. Coronary Blood Flow. In *Radioisotopes and Circulation*. Boston: Little Brown, pp. 126–135.
111. Schneider, R. A. 1972. In: *The Artery and the Process of Arteriosclerosis: Measurement and Modification*. S. Wolf (ed.) New York: Plenum Press, pp. 235–236.
112. Wolf, S. (ed.). 1972. *The Artery and the Process of Arteriosclerosis: Measurement and Modification*. New York: Plenum Press, pp. 228–235.
113. Friedman, M., and Rosenman, R. 1959. Association of specific overt behavior pattern with blood and cardiovascular findings. *JAMA*, 169:1286.
114. Bruhn, J. G., Paredes, A., Adsett, C. A., and Wolf, S. 1974. Psychological Predictors of Sudden Death in Myocardial Infarction. *Journal of Psychosomatic Research*, 18:187–191.
115. Bruhn, J. G., 1967. Social factors and coronary heart disease. *Journal of the Oklahoma State Medical Association*, Feb, 65–70.
116. Sussman, M. B. 1972. Family, kinship and bureaucracy. In *The Human Meaning of Social Change* ed. A. Campbell, and Converse, P.E., New York: Russell Sage Foundation.
117. Gibbon, E., 1827. *The History of the Decline and Fall of the Roman Empire*, vol. 1, p. 318. Oxford: Tallboys and Wheeler.
118. Hernandez-Peon, R., Sherrer, H., and Jouvet, M. 1956. Modifications of electrical activity in cochlear nucleus during "attention" in unanesthetized cats. *Science*, 123:331.
119. Locke, J. 1690. *An Essay Concerning Human Understanding*. In 4 books. London.
120. Gassendi, P. 1971. Syntagma philosophicum. In Fellows, O. E., and Torrey, N. L., (eds.) *An Anthropology of 18th Century French Literature*. 2nd ed., New York: Appleton-Century-Crofts, p. 6.
121. Bernard, C. 1926. *An Introduction to the Study of Experimental Medicine*. New York: Macmillan.
122. Richet, C. 1900. *Défense, fonctions de Dictionnaire de Physiologie*, vol. 4, p. 724, Paris: Baillière.

123. Cannon, W. B. 1925. Physiological regulation of normal states some tentative postulates concerning biological homeostatics. In: C. Richet, Ses Amis, ses colleques, ses elves- Auguste Pettit, ed., Medical Library, pp. 91.
124. Ratcliffe, H. L. 1964. Myocardial infarction: a response to social interaction among chickens. *Science* 144:425–426.
125. McKissick, G. E., Ratcliffe, H. L. and Koestner, A. 1968. Enzootic toxoplasmosis in caged squirrel monkeys *Saimiri sciureus. Pathologia Veterinaria* 5:538–560
126. DuBos, R. 1953. The germ theory revisited. Lecture delivered at Cornell University Medical College, New York, 18 March.
127. Pasteur, L. 1932. Compton, Piers. The Genius of Louis Pasteur, pp: 260–263, New York: MacMillan.
128. Rothlistberger, F. J., and Dickson, W. J. 1939. *Management and the Worker: An Account of a Research Program Conducted by the Western Electric Co.*, Hawthorne Works, Chicago Cambridge: Harvard University Press.
129. Spitz, R. 1974. *Grief: A Peril in Infancy.* New York: New York University Film Library. Film.

Index of Proper Names

Subject Index

For Product Safety Concerns and Information please contact our EU
representative GPSR@taylorandfrancis.com Taylor & Francis Verlag GmbH,
Kaufingerstraße 24, 80331 München, Germany

Printed and bound by CPI Group (UK) Ltd, Croydon, CR0 4YY
01/05/2025
01858612-0001